Understanding and Treating Cognition in Schizophrenia: A Clinician's Handbook

PHILIP D HARVEY PhD
PROFESSOR OF PSYCHIATRY
MT. SINAI SCHOOL OF MEDICINE
NEW YORK
USA

TONMOY SHARMA
CLINICAL NEUROSCIENCE RESEARCH CENTRE
STONEHOUSE HOSPITAL
DARTFORD
KENT
UK

MARTIN DUNITZ

© 2002 Martin Dunitz Ltd, a member of the Taylor & Francis group

First published in the United Kingdom in 2002 by Martin Dunitz Ltd, The Livery House, 7-9 Pratt Street, London NW1 0AE

Tel: +44 (0) 20 7482 2202
Fax: +44 (0) 20 7267 0159
E-mail: info@dunitz.co.uk
Webiste: http://www.dunitz.co.uk

A CIP record for this book is available from the British Library.

ISBN 1 84184 133 1

Although every effort has been made to ensure that all owners of copyright material have been acknowledged in this publication, we would be glad to acknowledge in subsequent reprints or editions any omissions brought to our attention.

Distributed in the USA by
Fulfilment Center
Taylor & Francis
7625 Empire Drive
Florence, KY 41042, USA
Toll Free Tel.: +1 800 634 7064
E-mail: cserve@routledge_ny.com

Distributed in Canada by
Taylor & Francis
74 Rolark Drive
Scarborough, Ontario M1R 4G2, Canada
Toll Free Tel.: +1 877 226 2237
E-mail: tal_fran@istar.ca

Distributed in the rest of the world by
ITPS Limited
Cheriton House
North Way
Andover, Hampshire SP10 5BE, UK
Tel.: +44 (0)1264 332424
E-mail: reception@itps.co.uk

Composition by Wearset Ltd, Boldon, Tyne and Wear
Printed and bound in Great Britain by The Cromwell Press, Trowbridge.

Contents

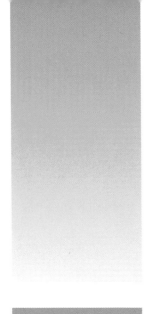

Acknowledgements

The research by Dr Harvey was supported by a Mental Health Clinical Research Center grant to Mt. Sinai School of Medicine and by the Department of Veterans Affairs VISN 3 Mental Illness Research, Education, and Clinical Center. The Janssen Research Foundation and the Lilly Research Foundation provided additional research support. Dr Harvey would like to thank the thousands of schizophrenic patients who have generously contributed their time to assist in the understanding and treatment of their illness. Without the contributions from patients and their carers, this research would be impossible.

The research by Dr Sharma was supported by the Wellcome Trust, The Stanley Foundation (USA), The National Lotteries Charity Board (UK), and National Alliance for Research in Schizophrenia and Depression (USA). Additional support was provided by Psychmed Ltd and the Janssen Research Foundation.

Introduction

This book describes the state of the art of our understanding of cognition in schizophrenia. We focus on a clear description of the types of problems seen, their importance, and how they can be treated. Our perspective is that cognition is one of most important, if not the most important, aspects of schizophrenic illness. We will try to prove this by a comprehensive evaluation of the most important aspects of cognition in schizophrenia, and by focusing on the clinical implications of these deficits for the everyday life of patients with schizophrenia. This book provides easy-to-follow, but sophisticated analyses of cognitive deficit, their implications, and newly developing strategies.

What is cognition?

High level cognitive functions are what separate humans from other primates. The intrinsically human activities of planning for the future, learning large amounts of complex information, and having elaborate and dynamic social relationships are dependent on these high level cognitive functions. Without these cognitive functions, the other intrinsically human activities are interfered with. In fact, schizophrenia is an illness involving impairments in planning, learning, and social activity that can be traced back to impairments in cognition.

Cognition can be referred to as all aspects of learning about, understanding, and knowing the world around oneself. Any object in the environment must be differentiated from the background, correctly identified, kept in mind, and then recalled at later points. In addition, solving problems, planning, and understanding complex verbal and conceptual material are important features of cognition as well. Terms like 'memory, attention, perception, and abstraction' are the words that psychologists use, sometimes confusingly and inconsistently, to describe the various mental processes that we consider cognition. As the rest of this book will demonstrate, impairments in these cognitive processes are probably the underlying cause of much of the well-known disability and dependency seen in patients with schizophrenia.

The organization of this book

In the first part of this book we will describe the types of cognitive deficits seen in schizophrenia. In so doing, we will also provide some of the fascinating history of the study of cognition in schizophrenia, followed by the evidence that cognitive deficits in the illness are an intrinsic part of schizophrenia and not caused by other aspects of the illness. Next we will describe the functional importance of these impairments. This includes the cost of the deficits, changes

with aging, and the direct clinical relevance, in real-world terms, of cognitive impairments. In addition, we show the latest evidence of changes in brain functioning that are associated with cognitive changes. We conclude the book with a discussion of the treatment of cognitive deficits. This is one of the areas where recent developments in research on schizophrenia are most promising and have the potential to change the overall outcome of schizophrenia. These sections of potential cognitive enhancement are in marked contrast to the history of negligible benefits of older treatments. Finally, the brain changes associated with cognitive enhancement in schizophrenia are also presented, with recent research demonstrating that treatments that improve cognition tend to normalize brain function as well.

This book has been written by two scientists whose specialization is the study of cognition in schizophrenia. It is based on our own perspective, which may be different from that of some others and may lead to differences in topical coverage and emphasis. This is also a short book, which does not provide the detail that longer texts and multi-author editions might. At the same time, we have tried to provide a reasonable selection of references to document our statements and provide sources for additional reading.

Philip D Harvey   **Tonmoy Sharma**
New York   **Dartford**

The history of cognition and schizophrenia

1

In the past 10 years there has been an explosion of interest in and research on cognition in schizophrenia. Anyone approaching this topic for the first time would think this interest and enthusiasm signified a recent discovery, such as the mapping of the human genome or understanding the newest developments in neurogenesis. However, the understanding that cognitive impairments are present in schizophrenia and even understanding of the specific domains of impairment dates back to the earliest descriptions of schizophrenia at the end of the 19th century.

Schizophrenia as we know it today originated in the clinical descriptions of Kraepelin (1919) and Bleuler (1950). Dementia praecox was Krapelin's descriptive formulation of schizophrenia, the term encompassing his developmental theory of illness. As a dementia, schizophrenia was conceptualized as a primary cognitive disorder, with onset early in adulthood and a progressive functional and intellectual decline present in most cases. Throughout his writings on the topic, Kraepelin described impairments in attention, motivation, learning, problem solving, and other cognitive skills. Equally salient in his formulation were the deficits in social functioning, independent living skills, and self-care ability that are now known to be a part of the impairments in functional capacity seen in patients with schizophrenia. Students of Kraepelin performed some of the first research on cognition in schizophrenia. Interestingly enough, the topics they studied, verbal skills and motor skill learning (referred to as procedural learning), remain the topics of extensive research today. Consequently, the centrally important research topics in cognition in schizophrenia have remained similar for the past 100 years.

Conceptions of schizophrenia: a history of controversy

When Bleuler re-named dementia praecox as schizophrenia, the term that is still in use, he did so partly to express a divergence of opinion with Kraepelin about a number of the issues involved in the conception of dementia praecox. Age of onset and the course of the illness were the two main areas of disagreement. Time has probably shown Bleuler to be correct in the idea that age of onset in schizophrenia is not restricted to early adulthood. Similarly, the idea that the illness inevitably progresses to a terminal state of dementia is also clearly not correct.

Yet, the areas of agreement between Bleuler and Kraepelin are of interest also. Bleuler divided the symptoms of schizophrenia into those that are seen as core features of the illness, referred to as

'fundamental' symptoms, and other secondary symptoms, referred to as accessory symptoms. The core features of the illness included impairments in the associative connections between thoughts and ideas, referred as 'loosening of associative threads'. Thus, Bleuler believed that deficits in critical cognitive processes were in fact the underlying cause of the central impairments in the illness, a splitting and loss of integrity of self.

Research following on from Blueler was based on the concept of deficits in associative connections. Some of the first studies on word associations examined the performance of patients with schizophrenia on single-word association tasks (Cat: _____) (Kent and Rosanoff, 1910). Later research in this area examined patterns of continuous responses to target association stimuli. Thus, Bleuler's theoretical perspective on the cause of schizophrenia was one of the factors leading to the use of word-association paradigms throughout psychiatry.

Many other aspects of cognition were studied during the early 20th century. Multiple studies focused on the performance of patients with schizophrenia on tests of intellectual functioning. By the mid-1940s enough research on cognitive functioning in schizophrenia had been published to allow for an extensive review paper (Hunt and Cofer, 1944), reviewing the first half-century of research on 'psychological deficit' in schizophrenia.

Controversies in the study of cognition

One of the controversies that developed in the early years of research on cognition in schizophrenia was whether patients with schizophrenia performed equally poorly on every test that they attempted, producing a global intellectual deficit, or had greater deficits in one or more critical aspects of functioning (Chapman and Chapman, 1973). This controversy is still ongoing. As will be seen in several of the later chapters, some researchers believe that the principal deficit in patients with schizophrenia is a massive impairment in all skill areas. Others believe that specific deficits in areas such as memory, attention, and problem solving are present and distinguishable from a backdrop of overall poor performance.

A second early controversy that has continued to the present day is whether certain cognitive deficits are characteristic of all patients with schizophrenia. Early and contemporary literature is full of references to schizophrenia as a disorder of attention, memory, abstraction, or other skills. The issue of whether every patient with schizophrenia has a specific deficit, like every patient with Alzheimer's disease has a memory deficit, is complex and is addressed in each of the following chapters.

There are important implications for the controversy regarding global versus specific deficits in cognition in schizophrenia. Impairments that were found to be present in every patient with schizophrenia might lead to important etiological implications. For example, if every patient had severe memory deficits, then the biological substrate of the memory system might be implicated in the overall etiology of schizophrenia. Conversely, global deficits mean that careful examination of multiple cognitive areas is required in patients with the illness, because if a patient performs poorly on any test that they are given, then the only areas of deficits that are not detected would be the ones that are not tested by the examiner. If patients with schizophrenia performed poorly on all tests administered, then the identification of 'specific' deficits would be suspect unless extremely comprehensive tests were administered and performance compared across all of the tests administered.

Another long-standing controversy in the area of cognition and schizophrenia is the approach that should be employed in assessment. The development of clinical neuropsychology as a professional discipline has led to several assessment traditions. The reliance on extensive understanding of normal performance, development of corrections for education, age, and other factors, and selection of cognitive domains based on understanding of the full range of normal cognition have resulted in studies that include extremely extensive assessment batteries

(Heaton et al, 1993). These batteries have the strength of the comprehensiveness and reliability and the limitations that they require highly skilled interpretation and not all patients with schizophrenia can comply with the assessment demands. Another limitation is that 'off the shelf' assessments may not be specifically relevant to the impairments seen in patients with schizophrenia.

In contrast, schizophrenia-oriented approaches, experimental in nature, have attempted to develop de novo cognitive assessments based on conceptions of the cognitive impairments seen in schizophrenia. While this method has the benefit of a close relationship of the cognitive assessments to the phenomenological processes of interest and ease of administration of this type of abbreviated assessment, these de novo instruments do not have normative standards that allow for a comprehensive comparison of the performance of patients to normal individuals. Furthermore, relative performance across cognitive domains cannot be measured in such a study. If patients have global performance deficits, then poor performance on a single assessment measure might be misinterpreted.

What did earlier research tell us?

Several important lessons have been learned from earlier research on cognition in

schizophrenia. Schizophrenic patients perform poorly on many measures of cognition, so any effective assessment must have several different measures. While the extent and coverage of a full neuropsychological battery may be a matter of debate, it is crucial to be able to identify whether any identified deficit is specific or part of a pattern of overall poor performance. This is referred to as identifying a 'differential deficit' (Chapman and Chapman, 1973). A second important development is the understanding that there is no specific deficit that is present in all patients with the illness. Such a 'pathognomonic' deficit has remained elusive, despite the interest of many researchers in identifying a deficit that might provide some underlying etiological unity in the wide-ranging diversity that is the phenomenology of schizophrenia.

Perhaps the most important lesson learned from the early research on schizophrenia is that cognitive deficits cannot be measured in isolation. Schizophrenia is a very diverse disorder, with wide variation in the presentation of positive, negative, and disorganized symptoms, functional outcome, and course of illness. Although Bleuler's theory of schizophrenia was that a cognitive deficit, a loosening of associative threads, was the underlying cause of the entire illness, there was very little specificity in prediction. Since Bleuler's time, the standards of scientific precision have increased considerably. The variability in symptoms across patients suggests no single deficit present in all patients could cause the notably diverse symptom presentation across patients.

One of the recent developments in research on cognition has been the design of research that has attempted to identify the correlation of cognitive deficits and other aspects of the illness (Neale et al, 1985). For instance, if it is believed that deficits in short-term memory interfere with the ability to plan speech, leading to formal thought disorder, a study must be designed that clearly tests this hypothesis. Comparing patients who have prominent thought disorder with those who do not on short-term memory tests would be an example of a test of this hypothesis (Harvey, 1985). Simply taking a sample of patients with schizophrenia, independent of their formal thought disorder status, and testing their short-term memory, would not be a suitable research design.

In the early years of research on cognition in schizophrenia, the failure to relate symptom status, whether positive, negative, or disorganized symptoms or functional deficits, to cognitive performance obscured the importance of cognitive functioning in the illness. If cognitive deficits were identified without reference to the behavioral referents of schizophrenia, their importance was relegated to academic interest. In contrast, the information presented later in this book shows that some of the cognitive deficits have notable clinical importance, particularly in the areas of prediction of functional status. Despite the identification of a whole array of cognitive impairments, earlier research did not fully elucidate their importance.

Summary

Most of the critical aspects of cognitive functioning in schizophrenia were identified in the first half of the 20th century. At the same time, research designs that did not identify the clinically important correlates of these deficits rendered the findings difficult to understand and not particularly relevant. It is important to understand that most cognitive deficits in schizophrenia were identified many years ago and that the study of cognition in schizophrenia is not a new development. What has evolved recently is a greater understanding of the importance of cognitive deficits, including their functional implications and their potential for influencing other aspects of the illness. An additional factor that reduced the impact of knowledge regarding cognitive deficits in schizophrenia is that for years it was believed that deficits on cognitive tests were caused by other aspects of the illness. This has been demonstrated to be untrue in the past few years, as reviewed in the next chapter.

It has become clear that understanding the characteristics of cognitive impairment in schizophrenia is only half of the story. Understanding what cognitive dysfunction does to the patient with schizophrenia, how it influences the quality of their life and their functioning in society, is the true clinical importance of research on cognition in schizophrenia. The next chapter shows the centrality of cognitive deficits to the syndrome of schizophrenia and the rest of this book illustrates the dimensions, importance, and treatment of these deficits.

References

Bleuler E. *Dementia praecox or the group of schizophrenias.* New York: International Universities Press, 1950.

Chapman LJ, Chapman JM. *Disordered thought in schizophrenia.* New York: Appleton, Century, Crofts, 1973.

Harvey PD. Reality monitoring in mania and schizophrenia: The association between thought disorder and performance. *J Nerv Ment Dis* 1985; **173**: 67–73.

Heaton RK, Grant I, Adams S. *Norms for an expanded Halstead-Reitan Neuropsychological Battery.* Odessa, FL: Psychological Assessment Resources, 1993.

Hunt JMcV, Cofer C. Psychological deficit. In: Hunt JMcV, ed. *Personality and behavior.* New York: Ronald Press, 1944, 971–1032.

Kent GH, Rosanaoff AJ. A study of associations in insanity. *Am J Insanity* 1910; **66**: 37–47.

Kraepelin E. *Dementia praecox and paraphrenia.* Edinburgh: E & S Livingstone, 1919.

Neale JM, Oltmanns TF, Harvey PD. The need to relate cognitive deficits and specific behavioral referents of schizophrenia. *Schizophr Bull* 1985; **11**: 286–91.

Cognitive deficits as a core feature of schizophrenia

2

Although cognitive impairments in schizophrenia have been described for years, there have always been lingering questions about whether these deficits reflect a central feature of the illness or whether they are a consequence of other aspects of the illness. After all, cognitive deficits are the result of performance on tests, which can conceivably be affected by many different factors. These factors include other symptoms of the illness, such as hallucinations or negative symptoms, treatment of the illness with antipsychotic medications, motivational factors, and global intellectual deficits associated with poor education or social deprivation.

As described in Chapter 1, Bleuler and Kraepelin both believed that cognitive deficits in schizophrenia were primary features of the illness and that, if there was a causal relationship between symptoms and cognitive deficits, cognitive deficits cause symptoms instead of the opposite. At the same time, schizophrenia was a less complex social problem during their time than it is now and the treatments offered were less diverse. It is conceivable that some of the manifestations of cognitive deficits are central to schizophrenia and other aspects are exaggerated by other components of the illness and its treatment. To explore this further, the following critical questions regarding the centrality of cognitive impairments in schizophrenia, will be examined.

Critical questions regarding the centrality of cognitive deficits

- Is poor cognitive performance caused by positive symptoms?
- Is poor cognitive performance caused by medication treatment?
- Is poor cognitive performance caused by poor motivation?
- Is poor cognitive performance caused by negative symptoms?
- Is poor cognitive performance caused by global intellectual deficits?

There exists a considerable amount of scientific research that addresses these issues. With some exceptions, the results of these studies suggest that cognitive impairments are remarkably unaffected by other confounding factors and indicate that cognitive impairment can be measured with considerable accuracy and validity.

Cognitive impairment is not caused by positive symptoms

It is a common belief in clinical practice that patients with schizophrenia are impaired in their cognitive functioning as a consequence of positive symptoms, such as auditory hallucinations. It seems logical to reach this conclusion because patients may have a tendency to respond to internal stimuli or to be preoccupied with their delusional beliefs. In this situation it appears as if the patient with schizophrenia cannot pay attention to their social environment or to the demands associated with cognitive testing. It is commonly said 'Why shouldn't patients with schizophrenia have attentional problems, after all, they are listening to those voices'.

The majority of the evidence, however, paints a picture that is quite different from this point of view. It has been found, for example, that the severity of auditory hallucinations and other positive symptoms in patients with schizophrenia are not correlated with the severity of their impairments in cognitive functioning measured by various neuropsychological tests (Addington et al, 1991; Davidson et al, 1995). Some patients may be untestable as a result of their positive symptoms, but those patients who are testable often have extremely severe positive symptoms. We also do not know how many normal individuals would refuse testing of the type offered to patients with schizophrenia. In the practice of clinical neuropsychology, for example, many patients with head injuries refuse testing as well.

Even more convincing, however, are the

results of studies that evaluate the same patient when they are psychotic and then again when they are not. These studies have found that impairments in memory and attention are very similar when the patients are tested while psychotic and then later when in remission from their symptoms (Harvey et al, 1990; Nuechterlein et al, 1986). If the same patient has the same level of cognitive impairment while actively hallucinating and later when they are not, the hallucinations, which vary in their severity, cannot be causing a stable cognitive deficit.

Furthermore, many different studies have demonstrated that cognitive deficits, in the areas of attention (Cornblatt et al, 1999), intellectual functioning (Davidson et al, 1999), and short-term memory (Harvey et al, 1981), are present in individuals before they develop signs of schizophrenia. If these deficits are present before the onset of psychosis, then there is no chance that they are caused by the experience of psychotic symptoms. As a result, cognitive impairments are present before, during, and after the occurrence of positive symptoms such as hallucinations. Their severity is also not related to the severity of the hallucinations or other positive symptoms. While severe positive symptoms may render some patients untestable, the research on testability of schizophrenic patients suggests that around 90% are fully testable by competent testers (Harvey et al, in press). This compares favorably to the results of

assessments of patients with head trauma or dementia.

Poor performance is not caused by medication treatment

It also is a common belief that neuroleptic medication is the cause of poor cognitive performance. This is understandable, because conventional antipsychotic medications have the potential to induce significant side effects. At the same time, there is very little evidence that this idea is true. The empirical literature suggests that, in fact, typical neuroleptic medication has essentially no impact on the majority of important cognitive functions in schizophrenia (Blyler and Gold, 2000; Medalia et al, 1988; Spohn and Strauss, 1989). One exception is the domain of motor skills, which appear to be slightly impaired by treatment with typical neuroleptic medication (Blyler and Gold, 2000). A limited subset of attentional measures is also influenced by traditional neuroleptic treatment (Oltmanns et al, 1979; Serper et al, 1994) and all of these measures are improved by this treatment.

There are two additional areas of evidence suggesting that antipsychotic medication could not be the principal cause of cognitive impairments. The first is historical. Cognitive impairment in schizophrenia was thoroughly described and studied before the introduction of antipsychotic medications. As noted in the first chapter, a comprehensive understanding of the characteristics, if not the importance, of cognitive impairments was well developed before the introduction of antipsychotic medications in the 1950s. Results of research conducted 50 years before antipsychotic medications could not be influenced by those medications.

There is contemporary evidence that suggests that patients who have never taken antipsychotic medications perform similarly on cognitive tests to patients who have been treated with them for several years. Several independent studies have confirmed that neuroleptic-naïve patients manifest a profile and severity of cognitive deficits that is consistent with that seen in patients with a history of treatment for several years (Bilder et al, 1992; Hoff et al, 1999; Saykin et al, 1994). These data also suggest that poor performance is not a consequence of treatment with antipsychotics, as well as demonstrating that treatment with these medications for several years does not normalize performance to any noticeable extent, on average.

This is some suggestion, however, that novel antipsychotic medications may actually increase schizophrenic patients' speed of information processing, information processing capacity, and psychomotor speed. The initial findings are reviewed in Chapter 12; it is still too soon to draw any conclusions with great certainty.

Cognitive deficits are not caused by poor motivation

Many of the classic descriptions of schizophrenia discuss poor motivation, lethargy, and other signs of reduced interest in and effort applied to social and occupational success. These motivational deficits are also described in terms of low levels of sensitivity to interpersonal feedback, leading to reduced need for social reinforcement. As a result, many believe that poor motivation is the cause of poor cognitive performance. There are several reasons to believe that this is not true.

First, clinical ratings of amotivation do not correlate with poor cognitive performance (Harvey et al, 1996). Second, the performance of patients with schizophrenia is consistent with their premorbid levels of functioning on several different cognitive tests. For example, the ability to read is consistent with premorbid educational attainment (Harvey et al, 2000); the ability to recognize information previously presented to them is also often unimpaired, while the ability to recall this information without prompts or cues is grossly impaired (Paulsen et al, 1995). Finally, intellectual performance, particularly in the area of verbal IQ, is much less impaired than other aspects of cognitive performance such as attention and memory (Gold et al, 1992). As a result, differential deficits can be identified. A single explanation, such as lack of appropriate effort while being tested, cannot simultaneously explain normal and impaired performance across different cognitive measures.

Furthermore, some research has indicated that patients with schizophrenia can improve their performance on certain cognitive tests with instruction (Green et al, 1992). If patients' poor performance was caused purely by motivational deficits, why would they want to improve their performance by co-operating with lengthy instructional procedures? It is more likely that some patients who are experiencing an extended session of failure during a testing session may refuse to continue. This is not a generic motivational deficit – it is a very normal human reaction to continuous feedback about poor performance.

Cognitive deficits are related to, but not caused by, negative symptoms

Measures from many different domains of cognitive functioning are more likely to be associated with the severity of negative symptoms than with the severity of positive symptoms (Addington et al, 1991; Addington 2000). One explanation for these results is that poor performance on cognitive tests is a function of negative symptoms and that the two constructs are essentially indistinguishable. There is overlap in the definitions of cognitive and negative symptoms. Some clinical rating systems for

negative consider deficits in abstract thinking and stereotyped thinking, clearly cognitive processes, to be negative symptoms (e.g. the Positive and Negative Syndrome Scale, PANSS; Kay, 1991). It is not surprising that the overall severity of negative symptoms would correlate with cognitive performance in such a rating system. Similarly, cognitive functioning is related to social and occupational performance, as described in Chapter 7. Some negative symptoms rating scales (e.g. the Scale for Assessment of Negative Symptoms, SANS;, Andreasen, 1983) consider these functional deficits to be negative symptoms, also leading to a high correlation between cognitive and negative symptoms. Other research, however, has shown that there is a gradient of correlation between negative and cognitive symptoms. Blunted affect is least strongly correlated with cognitive performance (Blanchard et al, 1994), while alogia, social, and occupational deficits are more strongly correlated (Harvey et al, 1996; 1997).

It is possible to distinguish negative and cognitive symptoms in other ways as well. In recent longitudinal research, it has been demonstrated that the severity of cognitive and negative symptoms are correlated with each other at successive assessments, but they do not show the patterns of correlation over time that would suggest a causal relationship (Harvey et al, 1996). Also, when patients are referred from long-term psychiatric care to community residences, their negative symptoms improve or remain stable but their cognitive impairments remain stable or worsen (Leff et al, 1994). This suggests that negative symptoms may be more reactive to generalized environmental and social situations than the severity of cognitive symptoms, which appear more intractable. The lack of differentially strong relationships between clinical measures of amotivation, compared to other aspects of negative symptomatology, also argue against a simple amotivation hypothesis.

The true nature of the link between negative and cognitive symptoms is still being studied. Further research may shed more light on the nature of the relationship between these correlated, but not identical, aspects of symptomatology.

Poor cognitive performance is not caused by global intellectual deficits

A well-replicated finding in the research literature is that patients with schizophrenia perform poorly on many different measures of cognitive functioning. As a result, it has been known for the past three decades that simply studying a single cognitive process does not allow for definitive statements about the importance of that process, because there is no guarantee that poor performance is not a function of a generalized deficit (see Chapter 1

for a discussion). The 'differential deficit' strategy, similar to the neuropsychological conception of a 'double dissociation', has been recommended as a partial solution (Chapman and Chapman, 1973). In this strategy, tasks are identified on which healthy individuals perform equivalently while schizophrenic patients perform relatively worse compared to normal individuals on one task but perform as well as the healthy sample on the other task. Many studies have shown that schizophrenic patients demonstrate differential deficits on tasks measuring visual and auditory information processing, verbal skills, and working memory. Differential deficits have also been identified within patients with schizophrenia. For example, it has been demonstrated that patients with schizophrenia performed relatively more poorly compared to healthy controls on tests of memory functioning than on measures of intellectual functioning (Gold et al, 1992). Similar results have been obtained when indices of premorbid skills such as reading as compared to current performance on other cognitive measures (Harvey et al, 2000).

It is also important to keep in mind that patients with schizophrenia vary widely in their premorbid and current intellectual functioning. Some patients with schizophrenia have evidence of intellectual decline relative to pre-illness levels, but others do not (Goldberg et al, 1993). Patients whose current IQ scores are consistent with their pre-illness functioning still have notable cognitive deficits in the areas of abstraction and problem solving (Weickert et al, 2000). This finding suggests that the presence of cognitive impairment in schizophrenia operates independently of overall intellectual intactness.

Other practical issues

In the assessment of any impaired population, there are also practical aspects of cognitive testing that can affect the validity of the results. If impaired performance is an artifact of problems with the testing, then the results may be invalid. In general, tests can only be valid if they are reliable and produce the same scores when administered repeatedly and if they are sensitive to factors that affect cognition in the general population such as age and education.

Much research on cognition in schizophrenia has demonstrated that it is possible to develop tests that have high stability over time. Patients with schizophrenia improve less with practice than normal individuals (Blyler and Gold, 2000), so assessment of patients with schizophrenia is less vulnerable to these artifacts than assessment of normal individuals. Older patients with schizophrenia and less educated patients perform more poorly, similar to what is typically found in normal individuals (Davidson et al, 1995; Harvey et al, 1998).

Thus, many of the practical requirements for assessment of these patients can be met.

The importance of cognitive impairment in schizophrenia

Since cognitive impairment is now known to be an independent and prominent feature of schizophrenia, its importance in the illness requires careful consideration. In contrast to many other disorders defined on the basis of specific types of cognitive impairment, such as delirium or dementia, general or specific cognitive deficits are not part of the diagnostic criteria for schizophrenia in Diagnostic and Statistical Manual of Mental Disorders (DSM) or International Classification of Diseases (ICD) criteria. In order to obtain approval for medication to be approved by the Food and Drug Administration (FDA) for the treatment of schizophrenia there are no requirements for demonstration of treatment efficacy for cognitive impairment or even a requirement to demonstrate that the medication does not worsen cognitive functioning.

How common is cognitive impairment in schizophrenia?

Although there has been little comprehensive research on this topic, some recent data suggest that cognitive impairment may be more common than most other symptoms of the illness. Most studies of cognitive functioning in schizophrenia have either considered a limited subset of cognitive measures or have not examined patients on a case by case basis. On a group-mean basis, patients with schizophrenia perform neuropsychological tests on average at the 2nd to 15th percentile (Harvey and Keefe, 1997), which would be considered impaired to borderline by most standards. In a recent study using case by case examination, it was demonstrated that only 30% of patients with schizophrenia would be considered neuropsychologically 'normal' (Palmer et al, 1997). While 70% of patients with schizophrenia were designated to be impaired on the basis of a comprehensive neuropsychological assessment, 5% of a sample of normal comparison subjects were seen to be abnormal.

The high prevalence of cognitive impairment in this study may even be reduced by the characteristics of the subjects studied. The sample in this study was largely high-functioning outpatients living in the community, who might be expected to have less cognitive impairment than poorer outcome patients. In a study of geriatric chronically hospitalized patients with schizophrenia (Davidson et al, 1995), 70% were found to fully meet concurrent criteria for dementia as well as schizophrenia, while the average mini mental state examination (MMSE) score in the sample was only 14.5

and only 5% did not meet criteria for 'questionable' dementia. The actual prevalence of cognitive impairment in schizophrenia across all of the variation in outcome is likely to be somewhere between these two estimates.

When the prevalence of other symptoms of schizophrenia is examined comprehensively, hallucinations, delusions, communication disorders, and negative symptoms are found to affect between 25% and 50% of patients with schizophrenia (Andreasen, 1983; 1984). The only symptom of schizophrenia that has been reported to have a higher prevalence than cognitive impairment is that known as 'lack of insight' or 'unawareness of illness' (Amador et al, 1991; World Health Organization, 1973). Although not a symptom of schizophrenia that is included in DSM-IV, unawareness of illness may itself be a sign of cognitive dysfunction (Young et al, 1993).

How severe are cognitive deficits?

As noted above, patients with schizophrenia often perform at low levels compared to healthy individuals. More importantly, patients with schizophrenia perform very poorly compared to patients with neurological and degenerative disorders. They have poorer global cognitive performance than patients who have suffered closed head trauma (Temkin et al, 1999) and poorer memory and conceptual performance than patients with focal epilepsy in the temporal and frontal lobes (Gold et al, 1994). They have worse memories than patients with chronic alcoholism (Allen et al, 1999) and learn information at the same rate as patients with Alzheimer's disease (Davidson et al, 1996). When neuropsychiatric conditions that are defined in terms of cognitive impairments are compared to patients with schizophrenia, the schizophrenic patients are often equally cognitively impaired.

There is nothing subtle about these deficits and the only way to miss them is to not look for them. Detailed cognitive assessments, as described in later sections of the book, have clearly described these deficits. As a result, it is no surprise that other areas of functioning that require cognitive skills, such as independent living and occupational functioning, are impaired as well. These issues are addressed in detail in later sections of the book.

What are the relative levels of impairment?

Table 2.1 presents the relative levels of severity of impairment across different cognitive ability areas. These deficits are presented in terms of the average across all patients, including those with very severe and less severe overall functional deficits. The severity columns, mild, moderate, and severe, are indexed in terms of relative impairment compared to healthy individuals of the same age and educational status. Mild is defined as performing less than 1 standard deviation below the normal mean, around the 15th percentile or less. Moderate reflects deficit levels up to 2 standard deviations below the mean, around the 3rd to 5th percentile.

Table 2.1
The severity of cognitive deficits in schizophrenia

Mild	Moderate	Severe
Perceptual skills	Distractibility	Verbal learning
Recognition memory	Recall memory	Executive functions
Naming	Visuo-motor skills	Vigilance
	Working memory	Motor speed
		Verbal fluency

Severity is measured as number of standard deviations (SD) below the mean for normal subjects (mild = 0.5–1 SD; moderate = 1–2 SD; severe = 2–5 SD)

Severe deficit areas are performed at the 1st percentile of the total distribution or worse. As can be seen in the table, learning, problem solving, and attentional functions are severely impaired, while naming and recognition memory are mildly impaired. Between these levels of impairment are delayed recall and selective attention, which are both moderately impaired on average.

While these levels of impairment are dependent on a number of different factors, especially the chronicity of the patients, they provide information about the importance of these deficits. In the next section of the book, these different aspects of cognitive functioning will be described in detail, including the specific substrates of the brain that are responsible for these impairments. In the final sections of the book, the functional implications and treatment strategies for these deficits will also be evaluated.

Conclusions

Cognitive deficits are central aspects of schizophrenia and are not caused by other features of the illness. These deficits are typically quite severe and consistent with the level of impairment seen in serious brain trauma and degenerative conditions. These impairments can be assessed accurately and interpreted validly. The implications of these deficits are clinically important and functionally meaningful.

The correlates and consequences of these impairments will be described in detail in the remainder of the book.

References

Addington J. Cognitive functioning and negative symptoms in schizophrenia. In: Sharma T, Harvey PD, eds. *Cognition in schizophrenia.* Oxford: Oxford University Press, 2000, 193–209.

Addington J, Addington D, Maticka-Tyndale E. Cognitive functioning and positive and negative symptoms in schizophrenia. *Schizophr Res* 1991; 4: 123–34.

Allen DN, Goldstein G, Aldarando F. Neurocognitive dysfunction in patients diagnosed with schizophrenia and alcoholism. *Neuropsychol* 1999; 20: 723–37.

Amador XF, Strauss DH, Yale SA, Gorman J. Awareness of illness in schizophrenia. *Schizophr Bull* 1991; 17: 113–32.

Andreasen NC. *The scale for the assessment of negative symptoms (SANS).* Iowa City, Ia: The University of Iowa, 1983.

Andreasen NC. *The scale for the assessment of positive symptoms (SAPS).* Iowa City, Ia: The University of Iowa, 1984.

Bilder RM, Lipshitz-Broch L, Reiter G. Intellectual deficits in first episode schizophrenia: evidence for progressive deterioration. *Schizophr Bull* 1992; 18: 437–48.

Blanchard JJ, Kring AM, Neale JM. Flat affect in schizophrenia: a test of neuropsychological models. *Schizophr Bull* 1994; 20: 311–25.

Blyler CR, Gold JM. Cognitive effects of typical neuroleptics: Another look. In: Sharma T, Harvey PD, eds. *Cognition in schizophrenia.*

Oxford: Oxford University Press, 2000, 241–65.

Chapman LJ, Chapman JP. *Disordered thought in schizophrenia.* New York: Appeleton-Century-Crofts, 1973.

Cornblatt B, Obuchowski M, Roberts S, Erlenmeyer-Kimling L. Cognitive and behavioral precursors of schizophrenia. *Dev Psychopathol* 1999; **11**: 487–508.

Davidson M, Harvey PD, Powchik P et al. Severity of symptoms in geriatric chronic schizophrenic patients. *Am J Psychiatry* 1995; **152**: 197–207.

Davidson M, Harvey PD, Welsh K et al. Cognitive impairment in old-age schizophrenia: a comparative study of schizophrenia and Alzheimer's disease. *Am J Psychiatry* 1996; **153**: 1274–9.

Davidson M, Reichenberg A, Rabinowitz J et al. Behavioral and intellectual markers for schizophrenia in apparently healthy adolescents. *Am J Psychiatry* 1999; **156**: 1328–35.

Gold J, Randolph C, Carpenter, CJ et al. Forms of memory failure in schizophrenia. *J Abnorm Psychol* 1992; **101**: 487–94.

Gold JM, Hermann BP, Randolph C et al. Schizophrenia and temporal lobe epilepsy. A neuropsychological analysis. *Arch Gen Psychiatry* 1994; **51**: 265–72.

Goldberg TE, Torrey EF, Gold JM et al. Learning and memory in monozygotic twins discordant for schizophrenia. *Psychol Med* 1993; **23**: 71–85.

Green MF, Satz P, Ganzell S, Vaclav JF. Wisconsin card sorting performance in schizophrenia: remediation of a stubborn deficit. *Am J Psychiatry* 1992; **149**: 62–7.

Harvey PD, Artioloa L, Desmedt G, Vester-Blockland E. Cross-national cognitive assessment in schizophrenia clinical trials: a feasibility study. *J Int Neuropsychol Soc*, in press.

Harvey PD, Docherty NM, Serper MR, Rasmussen M. Cognitive deficits and thought disorder. II. An eight-month followup study. *Schizophr Bull* 1990; **16**: 147–56.

Harvey PD, Howanitz E, Parrella M et al. Symptoms, cognitive functioning, and adaptive skills in geriatric patients with lifelong schizophrenia: a comparison across treatment sites. *Am J Psychiatry* 1998; **155**: 1080–6.

Harvey PD, Keefe RSE. Cognitive impairment in schizophrenia and the implications of atypical neuroleptic treatment. *CNS Spectrums* 1997; **2**: 41–55.

Harvey PD, Lombardi J, Leibman M et al. Cognitive impairment and negative symptoms in schizophrenia: a prospective study of their relationship. *Schizophr Res* 1996; **22**: 223–31.

Harvey PD, Lombardi J, Leibman M et al. Age-related differences in formal thought disorder in chronically hospitalized patients with schizophrenia: a cross-sectional study across nine decades. *Am J Psychiatry* 1997; **154**: 205–10.

Harvey PD, Moriarty PJ, Friedman J et al. Differential preservation of cognitive functions in geriatric patients with lifelong chronic schizophrenia: less impairment in reading compared to other skill areas. *Biol Psychiatry* 2000; **47**: 962–8.

Harvey P, Winters KC, Weintraub S, Neale JM. Distractibility in children vulnerable to psychopathology. *J Abnorm Psychology* 1981; **90**: 298–304.

Hoff AL, Sakuma M, Weineke M et al. Longitudinal neuropsychological follow-up study of first episode schizophrenia. *Am J Psychiatry* 1999; **156**: 1336–41.

Kay SR. *Positive and negative syndromes in schizophrenia.* New York: Brunner/Mazel, 1991.

Leff JP, Thornicroft G, Coxhead N, Trieman N. The TAPS Project. 22: A five-year follow-up of long stay psychiatric patients discharged to the community. *Br J Psychiatry* 1994; **165** (Suppl. 25): 13–17.

Medalia A, Gold J, Merriam A. The effects of antipsychotics on neuropsychological test results of schizophrenics. *Arch Clin Neuropsychology* 1988; **3**: 249–71.

Nuechterlein KH, Edell WS, Norris M, Dawson ME. Attentional vulnerability indicators, thought disorder, and negative symptoms. *Schizophr Bull* 1986; **12**: 408–26.

Oltmanns TF, Ohayon J, Neale JM. The effect of anti-psychotic medication and diagnostic criteria on distractibility in schizophrenia. *J Psychiatric Res* 1978; **14**: 81–91.

Palmer BW, Heaton RK, Paulsen JS, Jeste DV. Is it possible to be schizophrenic and neuropsychologically normal? *Neuropsychology* 1997; **11**: 437–47.

Paulsen TJ, Heaton RK, Sadek JR et al. The nature of learning and memory impairments in schizophrenia. *J Int Neuropsychol Soc* 1995; **1**: 88–90.

Saykin AJ, Shtasel DL, Gur RE et al. Neuropsychological deficits in neuroleptic naive patients with first episode schizophrenia. *Arch Gen Psychiatry* 1994; **51**: 124–31.

Serper MR, Davidson M, Harvey PD. Attentional predictors of clinical change during neuroleptic treatment. *Schizophr Res* 1994; **13**: 65–71.

Spohn HE, Strauss ME. Relation of neuroleptic and anticholinergic medication to cognitive functions in schizophrenia. *J Abnorm Psychol* 1989; **98**: 478–86.

Temkin NR, Heaton RK, Grant I et al. Detecting significant change in neuropsychological test performance: a comparison of four models. *J Int Neuropsychol Soc* 1999; **5**: 357–73.

Weickert TW, Goldberg TE, Gold JM et al. Cognitive impairments in patients with schizophrenia displaying preserved and compromised intellect. *Arch Gen Psychiatry* 2000; **57**: 907–13.

World Health Organization. *The international pilot study of schizophrenia.* Geneva: WHO, 1973.

Young DA, Davila R, Scher H. Unawareness of illness and neuropsychological performance in schizophrenia. *Schizophr Res* 1993; **10**: 117–24.

Learning and memory in schizophrenia

3

The human memory system is complicated and multifaceted. There are many components of this system, with many different ways to conceptualize memory performance. The common subdivisions of the system focus on both the type of information to be learned and remembered as well as the duration of storage of the information. Rather than provide detailed references for each of these domains of memory functioning, we recommend detailed texts. Lezak (1995) provides an excellent overview of the neuropsychological perspective on memory, while Tulving (1983) describes the entire episodic memory system in detail.

Different memory functions in schizophrenia range in the severity of their impairment from possibly the most impaired functions of all to the functions that demonstrate the least impairment. In this chapter we have chosen to describe each of the components of the memory system and then to describe the level of impairment in patients with schizophrenia.

Time-course of memory: the primary/secondary/long-term memory distinction

Some information is held in memory for relatively short periods of time and is then forgotten. A common example is recalling a phone number long enough to dial it or recalling driving directions long enough to execute a couple of simple operations (e.g. turn right at the next light and then look for the third road on the left). This type of memory function is referred to as short-term, primary, or working memory. This is such an important feature of schizophrenia that we have devoted the next chapter to it.

The process of learning information that is needed for longer-term use is referred to as secondary or declarative memory. Secondary memory encompasses the processes of acquiring new information with exposure, such as attending a college class or listening to instructions on how to perform tasks that constitute the core of your job. Another example is that of learning co-workers' or acquaintances' names after hearing them once or twice. This information can be either verbal or visuo-spatial in nature. The key component of secondary memory is that the information learned must be retrieved, often repeatedly, for adaptive use later. While it may be useful to forget phone numbers that are dialed only one time, it is an adaptive deficit to be unable to learn the names of your co-

workers or the address of your health care professionals.

Among the critical components of the process of learning new 'secondary' or 'declarative' memory information is the ability to encode information for storage and later use. Information is more easily encoded if it is somewhat familiar to the individual, but encoding can be hindered if new information is too similar to previously learned information. The process of getting information out of storage so it can be used later can be referred to as 'retrieval'. This includes both the ability to recall information spontaneously (e.g. 'tell me all of the words that I just read you') and the ability to recognize information previously heard and to distinguish it from information that was not previously presented (e.g. 'which 10 of these 20 words did I just read you?'). An additional feature of the retrieval system is its responsivity to cues. Examples of cued recall could include semantic cues ('Tell me all of the spices in the list'), phonological cues ('The word you are trying to remember rhymes with "hairs" '), or orthographic cues ('complete this word': Thr_ _d). Thus, declarative or secondary memory constitutes the highly important functions of encoding new information, remembering it after a delay, and being able to acquire and consolidate new learning.

Once information is thoroughly learned, it becomes part of the individual's long-term knowledge base. For example, information learned early in school, such as vocabulary or how to read certain words, is used over the course of the entire life without significant modification other than for updating on the basis of new information. The long-term storage for word meanings is often referred to as 'semantic memory'. Semantic memory includes both word meanings and their relationships to other words as well. Knowing both the meanings of 'cat' and 'dog' and that the two are members of several other hierarchical superordinate categories (pets, domestic animals, small animals, mammals, animals, living things, etc.) are examples of semantic memory.

Specialized memory systems

There are other memory systems that have importance for schizophrenia as well. Procedural memory refers to the ability to learn skills and motor acts that may not have a semantic underpinning. Learning how to sort items on the basis of appearance or to trace patterns are examples of procedural memory. Episodic memory refers to the memory for environmental and personal events. Remembering what happens over the course of a day and whether or not planned tasks have been completed would be an example of episodic memory, as would recalling that you had run into someone that you knew previously. Amnestic conditions are

characterized by marked deficits in episodic memory, wherein an individual with an amnestic condition cannot remember the events that occurred more than a few minutes previously. Interestingly, patients with amnestic conditions often have been spared procedural memory in the context of this completely impaired episodic memory (Squires and Zola-Morgan, 1996). Such findings, combined with the understanding of the types of lesions that impair procedural and episodic memory, have combined to lead to a better understanding of the brain systems involved in memory.

The brain substrates of memory functions

Different brain systems appear to be responsible for different memory functions. For instance, lesions of the medial temporal lobe, the diencephalon, the hippocampus, and associated midline structures appear to induce significant deficits in episodic and declarative memory systems (Gabrieli, 1998), while frontal lobe lesions are less likely to induce this type of impairment. Conditions causing deterioration of the basal ganglia are associated with deficits in procedural learning (Paulsen et al, 1995b). Impairments in semantic memory and the ability to utilize semantic strategies to facilitate memory appear to be induced both by lesions of the frontal lobe and by lesions in certain regions of the lateral temporal cortex. Results from neuroimaging studies have also suggested that activation of these brain regions is consistent with performance of tasks that are tapping these particularly memory systems. For instance, learning lists of words activates the medial temporal lobe and using the semantic memory system activates the lateral temporal cortex.

Memory impairments in schizophrenia

Patients with schizophrenia have wide-ranging and severe deficits in multiple memory functions, with these deficits being the most thoroughly studied aspect of cognition in schizophrenia. These deficits appear to be greater than would be expected on the basis of premorbid functioning, in that patients with schizophrenia routinely perform much more poorly on tests of memory functioning than would be expected on the basis of their premorbid intellectual functioning. Despite the fact that patients with schizophrenia often have reductions in their current intelligence compared to premorbid estimates (Weickert et al, 2000), patients with schizophrenia are typically found to perform more poorly on tests of certain aspects of memory functioning than their current IQ (Gold et al, 1992). Thus, memory functioning appears to be one of the aspects of cognition in schizophrenia with relatively greater impairment (Saykin et

al, 1991). Some aspects of memory in schizophrenia, however, appear to be relatively spared and to manifest modest to minimal impairments (Paulsen et al, 1995a). Finally, even within domains of memory functioning in schizophrenia (e.g. secondary memory), there appears to be a differential profile of deficit.

Impairments in secondary, declarative, or episodic memory

Types of impairments

This is the area of memory functioning where the greatest relative impairments can be detected. Patients with schizophrenia manifest a number of impairments on the input side in their memory functioning. When read a story or a list of words, they learn much less than healthy individuals (Saykin et al, 1991). If the list or story is repeated, they gain less information with repeated exposure than healthy individuals, showing a reduced 'learning curve' (Davidson et al, 1996). They are also less able to use semantic structure of information in order to aid their recall than healthy individuals (Harvey et al, 1986). Specifically, if a list of words contains information from a variety of different semantic categories (animals, fruits), healthy individuals are quite likely to report the information back in clusters, with the elements of different categories recalled adjacent to each other. Organized lists such as this are recalled more quickly and efficiently by healthy individuals. In contrast, people with schizophrenia do not tend to recall information in clusters and do not benefit from the embedded structure in lists in general. This is not simply a problem in not knowing to use this strategy, because even if they are told to cluster the information, they do not (Koh, 1978). Some have suggested (Aloia et al, 1996) that abnormalities in semantic structure are one of the most salient features of schizophrenia. Finally, this failure to benefit from structure is not due to some permanent abnormality in the semantic system, because if people with schizophrenia are exposed to strategies that force them to use the structure, such as having them sort the items into categories repeatedly and then recall them, their performance looks much more normal.

On the output side, patients with schizophrenia appear to recall less information than healthy individuals when they are asked simply to reproduce the information previously learned without cues or prompts (called 'free recall'; Paulsen et al, 1995a). This recall failure appears even when the reduced learning rate of patients with schizophrenia is accounted for. In contrast, the performance of most patients with schizophrenia on the ability to recognize information previously presented appears generally normal (Calev, 1984). For at least 50 years, this 'spared

recognition' memory phenomenon has been found repeatedly (Chapman and Chapman, 1973). Although most recognition memory tests are easier than free recall tests, even difficult recognition tests are performed relatively more normally (Calev et al, 1983). Finally, patients with schizophrenia are less able to benefit from prompted and cued recall than healthy individuals. However, this may be due to failures to encode the semantic features of words at the time of learning. When schizophrenic patients are exposed to manipulations to enhance semantic encoding at input, they are more responsive to cues at output.

Severity of deficits

Learning deficits in patients with schizophrenia are quite severe and consistent with those seen in dementia. Some have suggested that the impairment resembles anterograde amnestic conditions (Tamlyn et al, 1992). Several studies have compared patients with schizophrenia to patients with dementia caused by Alzheimer's disease and found that learning functions were very similar between the two groups (Davidson et al, 1996; Heaton et al, 1994). This level of deficit was similar across information that was presented only once (such as learning a paragraph) and several times (such as learning a word list in order to determine the learning curve). In terms of percentiles, patients with schizophrenia often learn at a rate that is two to three standard deviations below normative expectations. This is consistent with scores at the 1st to the 3rd percentiles of the normal distribution, which is the level of IQ scores of 55 to 70. These deficits appear generally consistent across verbal and visuospatial information (Putnam and Harvey, 1999), although there are difficulties in comparing performance on verbal and visual tests because of the fact that verbal information is usually much more familiar to individuals than the stimuli used in visual tests.

Deficits in recall appear to be somewhat less severe than learning deficits. Performance at delayed recall is often at the 5th to the 10th percentile of the normal distribution. Recognition memory is often performed at a level consistent with no impairment, relative to normative standards based on age and education. As a result, it can be concluded that deficits in the ability to learn new information are more profound than in the ability to reproduce that information later.

Symptom severity was initially suggested to be related to the severity of memory deficits. In reality, chronicity of illness appears more strongly linked to memory deficits. Several studies have shown that patients with more severe memory deficits were also more likely to have a chronic course of illness and to be treatment-refractory (Calev et al, 1983; Landro et al, 1993; Harvey et al, 1998). Thus, it may not be symptomatology as much as

lifetime functional outcome that correlates with poor anterograde memory functioning, an issue addressed in detail in Chapter 11.

Semantic memory

Types of deficits

There has been extensive debate regarding impairments in semantic memory, the memory system that stores word meanings and relationships between words. Research focusing on the structure of semantic memory in schizophrenia has typically used three different methodologies. These include studying word associations, studying priming effects, and studying the characteristics of structured verbal output. All of these methods have suggested that patients with schizophrenia have abnormalities in the way that their memory for semantic information is structured.

Word association studies are among the earliest research studies ever performed on patients with schizophrenia, dating back at least 90 years ago (Kent and Rosanoff, 1910). Results from these studies have indicated that patients with schizophrenia are more likely to produce unusual responses when presented with a single word stimulus and asked to produce the first word that comes to mind. These abnormal responses are more likely to be poorly linked to the dominant meaning of the word. For instance, if provided the word 'pen' most healthy individuals would likely say 'pencil', while a patient with schizophrenia may say 'sheep'. While this response seems quite strange, if one considers that a pen can be a fenced enclosure as well as a writing implement, the response is more understandable, but still unusual. More complex word association studies have provided multiple choice alternatives and demonstrated that patients with schizophrenia often provide responses that are poorly linked to the appropriate context of the word as presented.

Priming studies present the subject with a rapidly presented word stimulus (the prime) followed by a target letter string. For healthy individuals, the ability to tell if the second string is a word or a non-word letter string is facilitated by the prime being semantically related to the target word (top–bottom) and weakly facilitated by less strongly related words (teacher–school is faster than parent–school). In patients with schizophrenia, this priming relationship is weaker and there is less facilitation by the presentation of a highly related prime (e.g. Manschreck et al, 1988; Spitzer, 1997). These findings have been interpreted to suggest that the semantic network is either less well developed or less well interconnected in patients with schizophrenia than in healthy individuals.

Similar findings have been obtained from studies of the structure of verbal output

generated in various structured tasks. In verbal fluency tasks, subjects are often asked to produce a series of examples of a certain semantic category, like animals (Gourovitch et al, 1996). Studies of the sequence of the elements produced can provide inferences about the way the information in structured in storage. Patients with schizophrenia are much less likely than healthy individuals to produce output that follows a logical series of subsets of the overall category. For instance, healthy individuals often produce information in two general dimensions, such as wild–tame and large–small, with, for example, a series of large farm animals being produced in a group (cow, horse, donkey), followed by clusters of large wild animals (lion, tiger, bear). This structure is typically lacking from the output of individuals with schizophrenia, leading to the suggestion that the storage structure of semantic memory is impaired, above and beyond difficulties in access (Aloia et al, 1996). Furthermore, this impairment in the structure of semantic memory is hypothesized to underlie some of the problems that patients with schizophrenia demonstrate in terms of their ability to use semantic information to facilitate encoding of new information.

The severity of impairment

While many studies of semantic memory have used experimental tests without formal normative standards, studies using tests with norms indicate that semantic memory deficits are also in the range of the 3rd to the 5th percentile. Thus, deficits in access to semantic memory are severe and consistent with deficits in the ability to learn information, being greater than deficits in recall memory.

Procedural memory

Types of deficit

In contrast to the types of memory deficits described above, there is more controversy regarding the presence of procedural memory deficits in schizophrenia. Although some of the first research ever performed on cognition in schizophrenia, dating back to the 1890s examined performance on the pursuit rotor test, a procedural memory measure, some research finds only modest impairment in procedural memory in patients with schizophrenia. There has also been considerably less research on procedural learning in patients with schizophrenia than on declarative memory. At the same time, it is clear that patients with schizophrenia have evidence of deficits in the ability to learn motor skills. In contrast to the majority of patients with pure amnesic syndromes of cortical origin, patients with schizophrenia have evidence of slowed rates of motor learning and more motor errors than healthy comparison subjects (Kern et al, 1998).

One of the factors that confounds the assessment of procedural learning in schizophrenia is that, in contrast to other aspects of memory functioning, conventional antipsychotic treatment is known to have deleterious effects on procedural learning. Although this topic is discussed in much greater detail in Chapter 11, most measures of memory are relatively unaffected by treatment with conventional antipsychotic medications. Conventional medications blockade dopamine receptors in the basal ganglia, which is the region of the brain where procedural learning takes place. As a consequence, one of the effects of conventional antipsychotic treatment and consequential dopamine blockade, is that procedural learning has been reported to be poorer in patients treated with conventional medications than in those patients at baseline (Kumari et al, 1999).

Magnitude of deficits

The level of impairment in procedural learning is often not of the magnitude seen in studies of declarative memory. Patients with schizophrenia perform declarative memory procedures, on average, at levels consistent with about the 15th percentile of normal individuals, which is a much milder level of deficit than the other memory functions described above.

Long-term memory

Types of deficits

This is an important area of memory functioning, because it refers to the ability to adaptively employ information successfully learned previously. It is also an important area because this is the one aspect of the memory system with the most consistent evidence regarding preservation of functioning. Preserved functions in one aspect of memory, combined with impaired performance in other aspects, argues quite clearly against both motivational and global deficit explanations for the impaired performance. It can also inform the search for the neural basis of schizophrenia, because preserved versus impaired functioning may be occurring in different brain regions or in different connected brain systems.

Among the aspects of long-term memory that have received considerable attention in schizophrenia is that of academic skills learned while in school. Reading skills, in particular, have received this attention. The ability to recognize words, particularly those with irregular pronunciations, is a skill that is consistently associated with performance on intelligence tests (O'Carroll et al, 1992). Since these words were largely learned before the onset of schizophrenia, use of word reading ability to estimate premorbid intellectual functioning has been validated across several different studies. Even in patients with

evidence of cognitive and intellectual deterioration since the development of their illness (Harvey et al, 2000), reading is a skill area with notably less impairment and performance consistent with other benchmarks of premorbid functioning such as educational attainment.

Other aspects of earlier learning show evidence of very mild impairments. For instance, vocabulary and information measured with standard intellectual test methods are more impaired than reading scores in the same patients. These components of IQ tests require word definitions or informational responses to be provided verbally. Deficits in attention to verbally presented stimuli could impact performance, as could deficits in the ability to formulate coherent answers or impairments in the structure of semantic memory. As a result, some measures of earlier learning are potentially impacted by other factors, some of them outside the memory system and some of them components of the memory system.

There are other important implications of preserved earlier learning in the context of the very impaired ability to learn information described above in sections on declarative and episodic memory. Since the average patient with schizophrenia has grossly impaired new verbal learning in the context of a reasonably intact store of previously learned verbal information, there must be some change in memory performance at some time in the illness. Since this impairment in learning is not marked by lesions detectable at postmortem that are anywhere consistent with the notable lesions seen in amnesic conditions, the suggestion that this impairment in new learning is mediated by biochemical processes, rather than lesions or change in brain structure, is supported. This idea will be evaluated in more detail in the sections describing the treatment of cognitive deficits, particularly declarative memory, in Chapters 12 and 13.

Summary of relative memory deficits in schizophrenia

Figure 3.1 presents a graph of the relative severity of different types of memory deficits in schizophrenia. With 'normal performance' represented by 0 on the graph, the different levels of severity of impairment are presented as deviations from that score. Normal also takes into consideration the age and education of the subjects, since both notably affect memory performance. Quite clearly, one can see both the level of extreme deficit and the wide deviation across deficit areas in terms of the level of impairment.

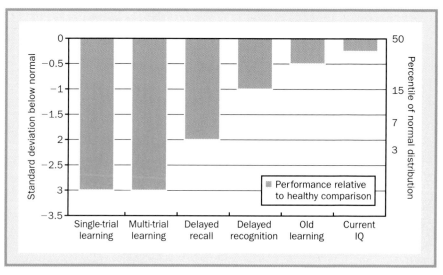

Figure 3.1
Relative memory deficits in schizophrenia.

The importance of memory deficits in schizophrenia

As described in Chapter 7, functional deficits in schizophrenia are intrinsically linked to deficits in cognitive performance, with memory deficits being one of the more consistent correlates. While this issue is reviewed in detail there, some information about the importance of memory in general will be provided.

Of all cognitive skills, impairments in declarative and episodic memory have the potential to be the most disabling. If one cannot remember ongoing events, one cannot update one's knowledge and proceed effectively from one activity to the next. In patients with Alzheimer's disease, progression of the inability to learn new information is the best predictor of functional disability (Green et al, 1993). These deficits in episodic memory have substantial impact on the ability to function adaptively.

Some institutionalized patients with schizophrenia manifest age disorientation. These patients misstate their own age by more than 5 years, indicating that they may have forgotten intervening events as well. This same group of patients is also likely to have disorientation to place, being unable to remember where they are even after lengthy stays in the same institution, often in the same ward (Harvey et al, 1995). On a more practical basis, the inability to recall everyday information makes independent living a challenge, because of the difficulties in planning typical activities. Furthermore, occupational efforts are challenged because the patient has an extremely difficult time learning the demands of a job and adapting flexibly to new information. Social deficits are also worsened by memory impairments, in that the inability to learn the names and other details regarding acquaintances impairs the ability to have meaningful social interactions with them.

In contrast to patients with Alzheimer's disease, patients with schizophrenia have an early onset of their memory deficits and spend their entire life with grossly impaired memory functioning. As described in Chapter 7, the adaptive implications of these memory deficits are quite profound. Much of the lifelong functional deficit in schizophrenia may be related, quite simply, to the fact that patients with schizophrenia have great difficulty learning new information. This deficit leaves them frozen in time and unable to change with new environmental, social, and personal demands.

Conclusion

Memory impairments in schizophrenia are wide-ranging and severe. They are probably the most severe impairment in patients with schizophrenia and have marked adaptive implications. A careful assessment of the parameters of memory deficits in schizophrenia leads to the several important insights regarding the course of cognitive deficits in schizophrenia, the role of motivation in cognitive performance, and possible brain regions that are affected and spared in the illness. We will return to our discussion of the importance of memory deficits later and will also discuss the latest attempts to treat them.

References

Aloia MS, Gourovitch ML, Weinberger DR, Goldberg TE. An investigation of semantic space in patients with schizophrenia. *J Int Neuropsychological Society* 1996; **2**: 267–73.

Calev A. Recall and recognition in chronic nondemented schizophrenics: the use of matched tasks. *J Abnorm Psychology* 1984; **93**: 172–7.

Calev A, Venables PH, Monk AF. Evidence for distinct verbal memory pathologies in severely and mildly disturbed schizophrenics. *Schizophr Bull* 1983; **9**: 247–64.

Chapman LJ, Chapman, JM. *Disordered thought in schizophrenia*. New York: Appleton, Century, Crofts, 1973.

Davidson M, Harvey PD, Welsh K et al. Cognitive impairment in old-age schizophrenia: a comparative study of schizophrenia and Alzheimer's disease. *Am J Psychiatry* 1996; **153**: 1274–9.

Gabrieli JDE. Cognitive neuroscience of human memory. *Annual Rev Psychol* 1998; **49**: 87–115.

Gold JM, Randolph C, Carpenter CJ et al. Forms of memory failure in schizophrenia. *J Abnorm Psychology* 1992; **101**: 487–94.

Gourovitch ML, Goldberg TE, Weinberger DR. Verbal fluency deficits in patients with schizophrenia: semantic fluency is differentially impaired as compared to phonological fluency. *Neuropsychology* 1996; **10**: 573–7.

Green CR, Mohs RC, Schmeidler J et al. Functional decline in Alzheimer's disease: a longitudinal study. *J Am Geriatr Soc* 1993; **41**: 654–61.

Harvey PD, Earle-Boyer EA, Wielgus MS, Levinson JC. Encoding, memory and thought disorder in schizophrenia and mania. *Schizophr Bull* 1986; **12**: 252–61.

Harvey PD, Lombardi J, Kincaid M et al. Cognitive functioning in chronically hospitalized schizophrenic patients: age-related changes and age disorientation as a predictor of impairments. *Schizophr Res* 1995; **17**: 15–24.

Harvey PD, Moriarty PJ, Friedman JI et al. Differential preservation of cognitive functions in geriatric patients with lifelong chronic schizophrenia: reduced impairment in reading scores compared to other skill areas. *Biol Psychiatry* 2000; **47**: 962–8.

Harvey PD, Powchik P, Mohs RC, Davidson M. Memory functions in geriatric chronic schizophrenic patients: a neuropsychological study. *J Neuropsychiatry Clin Neurosci* 1995; **7**: 207–12.

Harvey PD, Howanitz E, Parella M et al. Cognitive, adaptive and symptomatic features of schizophrenia in late life: a comparison of nursing home, chronically hospitalized and acutely admitted patients. *Am J Psychiatry* 1998; **155**: 1080–6.

Heaton RK, Paulsen JS, McAdams L-A et al. Neuropsychological deficits in schizophrenics: relationship to age, chronicity, and dementia. *Arch Gen Psychiatry* 1994; **51**: 469–76.

Kent GH, Rosanoff AJ. A study of associations in insanity. *Am J Insanity* 1910; **66**: 37–47.

Kern RS, Green MF, Marshall BD Jr et al. Risperidone vs haloperidol on reaction time, manual dexterity and motor learning in treatment-resistant schizophrenia patients. *Biol Psychiatry* 1998; **44**: 726–32.

Koh SD. Remembering of verbal materials by schizophrenic young adults. In: Schwartz S, ed. *Language and cognition in schizophrenia.* Hillsdale, NJ: Erlbaum, 1978, 59–99.

Kumari V, Somi W, Sharma T. Normalization of information processing deficits in schizophrenia with clozapine. *Am J Psychiatry* 1999; **156**: 1046–51.

Landro NI, Orbeck, AL, Rund BR. Memory functioning in chronic and non-chronic schizophrenics, affectively disturbed patients and normal controls. *Schizophr Res* 1993; **10**: 85–92.

Lezak MD. *Neuropsychological assessment* 3rd edn. New York: Oxford, 1995.

Manschreck TC, Maher BA, Milavetz JJ et al. Semantic priming in thought disordered schizophrenic patients. *Schizophr Res* 1988; **1**: 61–8.

O'Carroll RE, Walker M, Duncan J. Selecting controls for schizophrenia research studies: The use of the National Adult Reading Test (NART) as a measure of premorbid ability. *Schizophr Res* 1992; **8**: 137–41.

Paulsen JS, Heaton RK, Sadek JR et al. The nature of learning and memory impairments in schizophrenia. *J Int Neuropsychol Soc* 1995a; **1**: 88–99.

Paulsen JS, Salmon DP, Monsch A et al. Discrimination of cortical from subcortical dementias on the basis of memory and problem-solving tests. *J Clin Psychol* 1995b; **51**: 48–58.

Putnam KM, Harvey PD. Memory performance in geriatric and nongeriatric chronic schizophrenic patients: a cross-sectional study. *J Int Neuropsychol Soc* 1999; **5**: 494–501.

Saykin AJ, Gur RC, Gur RE et al. Neuropsychological function in schizophrenia: selective impairment in memory and learning. *Arch Gen Psychiatry* 1991; **48**: 618–24.

Spitzer, M . A cognitive neuroscience view of schizophrenic thought disorder. *Schizophr Bull* 1997; **23**: 29–50.

Squires LR, Zola-Morgan S. Structure and function of declarative and nondeclarative memory systems. *Proceedings of the American National Academy of Sciences* 1996; 13 515–22.

Tamlyn D, McKenna PJ, Mortimer AM et al. Memory impairment in schizophrenia: its extent, affiliations and neuropsychological character. *Psychol Med* 1992; **22**: 101–15.

Tulving E. *Elements of episodic memory.* NY: Academic Press, 1983.

Weickert TW, Goldberg TE, Gold JM et al. Cognitive impairments in patients with schizophrenia displaying preserved and compromised intellect. *Arch Gen Psychiatry* 2000; **57**: 907–13.

Working memory in schizophrenia

4

Working memory refers to memory for information that is briefly retained and used immediately in an adaptive manner. Referred to also as 'primary', 'immediate' or 'short-term' memory, working memory is the collection of processes that keep information in mind while it is needed and then either transfers it to the processes that prepare it for longer-term storage or discard it.

This working-memory information can be spatial, such as a location in the immediate visual field or it can be verbal, such as a telephone number. Working memory also retains information regarding the source of information in mind, such as 'Did someone tell me that idea or did I think of it myself?' Working memory may require rapid operations to be performed on the information held in mind, such as deciding which of three menu options is the least expensive or which of several phone numbers is the local number.

Working memory (types of information stored):
• spatial locations • object identity • sequence data • source of information • emotional connotation

Information in working memory is generally forgotten fairly soon after it is processed, indicating that forgetting is actually an adaptive function in regard to most of the information that people are exposed to on a daily basis. There is reason to believe that each and every one of these working memory functions, from the recall of a briefly presented spatial location to adaptive forgetting, is impaired in schizophrenia. Each of these working memory functions also has an important functional role, indicating that working memory deficits are among the most problematic cognitive impairments in schizophrenia.

The classic working memory model

The original theoretical model of working memory was produced by Alan Baddeley (Baddeley and Hitch, 1974). He hypothesized that there were two general components of working memory, brief storage systems (slave systems) and a central executive. Each slave system is hypothesized to be sensory modality-specific and limited in storage capacity, with a visual 'scratchpad' and a verbal 'articulatory loop' (Baddeley, 1986). These systems simply retain information without modification. The central executive is the system that manipulates the information retained in the modality-specific storage and also the system

that responds to changes in processing load by allocating other cognitive resources to handle fluctuations in load that would ordinarily exceed the capacity of each of the slave systems. Furthermore, the central executive makes decisions regarding which information can be allowed to be forgotten and which information is selected for additional processing and transfer into longer-term storage. Thus, in the Baddeley model there are various connected storage systems which are controlled and managed by higher-level control processes.

The relationship of executive functions and working memory

The Baddeley model demonstrates the intrinsic relationship between problem solving and cognitive allocation, the intrinsic core features of executive functioning, and working memory. It is impossible to solve problems or to select a strategy if the current environment and current cognitive operations cannot be kept immediately in mind and accessed upon demand. If an individual were to have a complete loss of working memory, that person would be unable to perform even the most simple executive tasks. Furthermore, the cortical localization of working appears similar to that of many executive functioning operations as well.

At the same time, executive functioning is

not identical to working memory and there are many working memory functions that have no discernable executive component. For instance, there is no executive component to the recall of a simple spatial location. Simultaneously, there are executive functions with little working memory component. It is important to realize that these are separate, but interdependent, scientific constructs and that determining that a patient has a deficit in working memory does not demonstrate an executive functioning impairment and vice versa. The next chapter on executive functions will provide even more information about the points of convergence and divergence of these two aspects of cognitive functioning.

The cortical localization of (some) working memory functions

One of the first identified brain-behavior relationships in neurobiology was the discovery that monkeys with massive lesions to the frontal lobes were unable to perform a simple 'delayed response task' (Jacobsen, 1936). In this task a hungry monkey is shown a raisin being placed into one of two cups in front of the animal. An opaque shield is then placed in front of the two cups for a delay period, after which the monkey reaches for one of the two cups. Thus the task simply requires memory for a spatial location. Frontal lobe lesions reduce performance on this task to chance levels. Humans with similar lesions also have deficits in working memory, with different regions in the frontal cortex producing different types of working memory deficits in simple two-alternative forced choice tasks. Dorsolateral lesions produce difficulties in delayed response, as described above. Orbitofrontal lesions produce deficits in object alternation (Oscar-Berman and Bonner, 1985). In object alternation, the task is to respond to the side opposite the location of the subject's prior response. So, if the last response was to the left, the correct next response is to the right. Lesions of both dorsolateral and orbitofrontal regions reduce performance on delayed alternation tasks. Delayed alternation tasks require the subject to respond to the location opposite the last correct response. So, if the last correctly located target was on the left, the next correct response will be to a target on the right.

Patients with schizophrenia have deficits in all three of these spatial working memory paradigms, with their greatest deficits being in delayed alternation and object alternation paradigms (Figure 4.1). While these findings have been sited as evidence for the contention that patients with schizophrenia have deficits similar to those individuals with frontal lobe lesions, there is no evidence of formal lesions in the frontal lobe in patients with schizophrenia. Other biological factors such as abnormal neurotransmitter activity, also

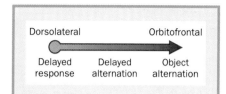

Figure 4.1
Frontal lobe lesions and the topography of working memory deficits.

investigated with working memory paradigms, are implicated in normal and abnormal working memory.

The neurotransmitters associated with working memory

Working memory is one of the extensively researched aspects of cognitive functioning in terms of cortical neurotransmitter determinants, largely because it can be measured online with animals. Extensive research performed in the laboratory of Patricia Goldman-Rakic has demonstrated that manipulations of cortical catecholamines, particularly in the anterior frontal cortex, influence working memory functioning. Using a spatial delayed response paradigm that measures eye movement responses to a visual target location in primates, it has been shown that a) there are individual neurons in the frontal cortex that are sensitive to specific spatial locations; and b) these neurons are sensitive to the influences of dopamine and norepinephrine. Administration of agonists to these transmitters (Arnsten et al, 1988; Sawaguchi and Goldman-Rakic, 1991) improves performance while antagonists (Arnsten et al, 1999; Sawaguchi and Goldman-Rakic, 1994) that reduce the activity of these transmitters reduce performance. Relatively similar effects have been produced in studies of both dopamine and norepinephrine, suggesting that both may be important determinants of working memory functioning. Treatment studies, reviewed in Chapter 13, have also suggested that drugs that increase norepinephrine (NE) activity improve spatial working memory in patients with schizophrenia.

There are two important scientific aspects of these findings. The first is that these memory functions were clearly localized to the frontal lobes in primates. Neurons responsible for the detection of the stimulus were located in posterior cortical regions, while the neurons that were active during memory retention were exclusively frontal in location (Williams and Goldman-Rakic, 1995). Given the long-time conceptualization of schizophrenia as a disorder of frontal lobe function, this evidence suggests that spatial working memory deficits may be an important index of some type of dysfunction of the frontal cortex. Chapter 10 presents information suggesting that patients with schizophrenia fail to activate their frontal lobes as extensively as healthy individuals while performing working memory tests. This under-activation may explain why frontal lobe dysfunction may exist in schizophrenic patients in the absence of postmortem evidence of lesions to that region of the cortex.

The second important aspect of these findings is of biochemical specificity. Dopamine has been a central feature of biological models of schizophrenia since the discovery of the mechanism of action of conventional antipsychotic medications. More recent conceptions of the pathology of schizophrenia focus more on regional dopaminergic abnormalities than on global overactivation of the dopamine system (Davis et al, 1991). Underactivity of cortical dopamine neurons has been a central model of cognitive deficit in schizophrenia in the past decade. Several lines of investigation have suggested underactivity or under-proliferation (Okubo et al, 1997) of cortical dopaminergic neurons and correlations between underactivity of these neurons and impairments in cognitive tasks thought to require frontal lobe involvement, including working memory (e.g. Daniel et al, 1991; Kahn et al, 1994). The indication of the intrinsic relationship of both dopamine and the frontal cortex in cognitive impairments that are commonly found in schizophrenia has drawn together much of the thinking of the past decade regarding regional brain dysfunction and schizophrenia.

Other types of working memory

There are other types of working memory deficits in schizophrenia. In fact, simple spatial delayed response tasks involve memory, without much of the working component. Many other aspects of working memory have been identified, and many of them are clearly impaired in schizophrenia.

Object working memory

Object working memory refers to visually-oriented working memory of objects in the visual field. If you see a complex stimulus situation, such as a street scene from London or New York and are required soon after to remember if you saw a blue car, this would be object working memory. This type of working memory may have a slightly different pattern of cortical localization than working memory for a simple spatial location (Wilson et al, 1993).

Memory span and manipulation tasks

Schizophrenic patients are not markedly impaired in simple measures of short term memory span (such as digit span), compared to their more severe deficits in secondary memory (Chapter 3), executive functioning (Chapter 5) and attention (Chapter 6). At the same time, patients with schizophrenia have been shown to have a short-term memory span of about one item less than healthy individuals (Gruzelier et al, 1988). Since healthy individuals have a memory span of about seven plus or minus two items, there are some potential adaptive consequences of even minor deficits. In North America, phone numbers have seven digits, and up to 10 if an area code has to be dialed. Western Europe typically has numbers of similar length. This number of digits evolved for a reason: it is typically within the memory span of most normal individuals. After all, the three-digit area codes in the US are so familiar that they can be recalled as if they were a single item. If you forget even one digit in a phone number, however, you get a wrong number. As a result, schizophrenic patients' 'mild' impairment, the typical inability to recall seven digits, can make it difficult for them to dial phone numbers and, importantly for many types of employment, to take phone messages. This is an area where a mild deficit may push the individual below the level of acceptable functioning.

In more complex span tasks, those with a large 'working' component, patients with schizophrenia have very severe deficits. For instance, if asked to listen to a list of scrambled numbers and letters, such as '5 G 3 A', and report them in ascending order, with the numbers followed by the letters, they often fail at items that are as short as this

example (Gold et al, 1997). In addition, when asked to perform serial addition tasks, such as successively adding together consecutive members of a series of numbers, such as '3' '4' '2', they are markedly poorer than healthy individuals.

Finally, a task that is routinely used in research involving neuroimaging of working memory is called the 'n-back' test. In this test, a subject sees a succession of stimuli, such as numbers, letters, or items in a predefined spatial location. After the presentation of each item, they are asked to respond with the item that occurred a specified numbers of items previously. For instance, '0-back' would involve responding to each item with its own identity. Since this task requires perception of the stimulus, but not memory, this is typically a control condition for more memory demanding conditions. For instance, a '1-back' condition would require the following responses to the following stimulus sequence:

| 1–2–5–6–2 | [Stimulus] |
| – 1 2 5 6 | [Response] |

A '2-back' condition would elicit the following responses:

| 1–2–5–6–2 | [Stimulus] |
| – – 1 2 5 | [Response] |

The use of this task has lead to the identification of one of the more intriguing findings on working memory in schizophrenia, one that has been replicated in slightly different format in studies of attentional functions. Reminiscent of their memory span, patients with schizophrenia perform very similarly to healthy individuals, at one less level of delay (Callicott et al, 2000). In other words, schizophrenic patients perform 1-back conditions like healthy individuals perform 2-back tests, while 2-back tests are performed like 3-back tests.

As described in Chapter 10, neuroimaging studies have also shown patterns of brain activation that are quite consistent with these performance patterns. Presented in greater detail in that chapter, it has been found that the brains of patients with schizophrenia performing under loads that can be managed by healthy individuals resemble the brain of these same healthy individuals performing under higher loads. Thus, the working memory performance, and concurrent brain functions, of people with schizophrenia, resembles a normal brain under overload conditions.

These findings suggest that patients with schizophrenia are operating under conditions that limit their processing capacity, but are not using strategies that are substantially different, from healthy individuals. The use of these simple manipulations of changing difficulty of processing demands has proven extremely informative in understanding the potential mechanisms of processing deficits in patients with schizophrenia. We will return to this issue in Chapter 10 where we discuss the brain changes associated with working memory dysfunctions in more detail and in Chapters 12 and 13 where we talk about the treatment of working memory deficits with antipsychotic medications and specific cognitive enhancing medications.

Source monitoring

When something is maintained in working memory, there are multiple informational components stored. In order for information to be used successfully, there are several different attributes of the information associated with it that are also retained. These components are contained in Table 4.1. As

Table 4.1
Characteristics of information stored in working memory

Stimulus modality	*Visual/auditory/other*
Verbal characteristics	*Verbal/nonverbal*
Generation status	*Self/other*
Emotional connotation	*Neutral/affective*

shown in this table, all information in short-term memory also carries information tags that allow for evaluation of the characteristics of the information. For instance ideas, action plans, and emotional reactions are tagged as self-generated and are then evaluated later as the products of the individual's conscious planning process.

Imagine that one could not determine if the information in your short term memory was an idea that you came up with or was something that you heard somewhere else. Sometimes, monitoring the status of this information is easy:

You think.

'That painting in front of me is the Mona Lisa.'

This is obviously an idea that came to mind on the basis of environmental information, including both the knowledge that you are in Paris and in the Louvre, the fact that you have seen this painting many times before, and the fact that the sign in front of the painting, although in French, identifies it as the Mona Lisa.

The situation where the problem comes up for schizophrenic patient is this one:

You are in a crowd, say, in the subway;

The idea comes into your mind 'You're dressed like a bum'.

You can't tell if someone nearby just said this to you (which is plausible, you don't have a job and your clothes are several years old).

Or

This idea came into you head because you personally are embarrassed about your clothes, which are, after all, several years old.

Monitoring the *source* of information in your mind is also a working memory function. Extensive research on working memory has focused on this issue in healthy individuals (Johnson and Raye, 1981; Johnson et al, 1993). There are multiple factors that influence accuracy of source monitoring in healthy people. For instance, self-generated information is most easily recognized. For example, if you tell someone a story, you are quite likely to remember that the information in your short-term memory is associated with the story that you told. If you see something and want to tell someone about it, most healthy individuals can determine if they have told the story yet, because their recollection of the situation is still sensory (I saw it) and not verbal (I heard it) and not generated (I told them about it).

Patients with schizophrenia do not show this 'generation effect'. If you can't tell if the information in your mind is an idea you had or is something that someone told you, then it is easy to get confused. If you get confused like this, you don't know if the idea that is currently in your mind is an idea or self-evaluation (I am a failure) or a perceptual experience coming from the environment.

This confusion between externally-generated information and self-generated information is crucial to several theories of the development of hallucinations and delusions in schizophrenia (Keefe, 2000). Monitoring of your experience (i.e. autonoetic processes) is a critical part of normal cognitive functioning. It helps distinguish external occurrences from internal experiences and, at its most basic level, helps to monitor current physical factors, such as location, movement, and body orientation. Several theorists have suggested that working memory failures in schizophrenia are similar to those seen in stroke patients (Keefe, 1998). Some of these patients have impairments in awareness of their ongoing environment that is so extreme that they will deny the existence of their own body parts, not to mention denying the contents of their conscious awareness of events that have recently occurred. Deficits in 'autonoetic awareness', sometimes referred to as 'autonoetic agnosia' (inability to recognize the contents of your consciousness) are commonly reported in schizophrenic patients and may be related to the presence of hallucinatory experiences. Thus, a subtype of working memory deficit may have major importance in the cause of some of the central symptoms of the illness. The significance of other aspects of working memory impairment, however, may be greater for the outcome of the illness.

The importance of working memory deficits in schizophrenia

Working memory deficits have clinical and functional importance at several different levels in the understanding of schizophrenia. Functionally, the inability to recall relatively modest strings of information has the potential to cause significant functional impairments. If you can't remember a telephone number, there are multiple sources of eventual potential social and occupational problems that would follow. Deficits in awareness of whether information in your memory came from your own mind or from somewhere else may be at the root of many of the positive symptoms of the illness. An inability to tell the difference between information that you heard and information that you imagined may be at the root of auditory hallucinations. Inability to tell the difference between information that you thought about telling someone else and information that you told them about may be related to communication impairments. If you thought about telling someone about an occurrence but never really did tell them, you might later refer to the information that you thought about as if it really had been presented to them. Many linguistic studies of the speech of patients with schizophrenia note that these individuals talk about many aspects of situational information as if they had been discussed before, even if they never were brought up overtly by the patient who is speaking (Harvey, 1985).

Working memory may also offer a key to some of the biochemical and functional brain abnormalities in schizophrenia. As noted earlier, abnormalities in catecholaminergic functions in the frontal cortex are associated with deficits in working memory, Later research will need to examine the specific relationship between normalization of the neurotransmitter or regional cortical functions and normalization of working memory. As shown throughout this chapter, working memory deficit is one of the areas of cognitive deficit that may have importance for understanding positive symptoms (i.e. hallucinations), disorganized symptoms (i.e. formal thought disorder), and functional impairments.

Conclusion

Working memory deficits in schizophrenia have both clinical importance and importance for the understanding of the etiology of the disorder. Since these impairments are present in schizophrenia, linked to specific symptoms, and have understandable biological and neuroanatomical correlates, they have the potential to provide a 'clinical laboratory' for the understanding of the illness. While these impairments are clearly not the only underlying impairment in the disorder and do

not explain all other aspects of cognitive impairment, they are among the cognitive deficits with the most widely understood biological and neuroanatomical basis. As a result, study of the treatment of these impairments may provide broad insights into the biology of schizophrenia and the treatment of other aspects of the illness.

References

Arnsten AFT, Cai JX, Goldman-Rakic PS. The alpha-2 adrenergic agonist guanfacine improves memory in aged monkeys without sedative or hypotensive effects: evidence for alpha-2 receptor subtypes. *J Neurosci* 1988; **8**: 4287–98.

Arnsten AFT, Mathew RJ, Ubriani R et al. Alpha-1 noradrenergic receptor stimulation impairs prefrontal cortical cognitive function. *Biol Psychiatry* 1999; **45**: 26–31.

Baddeley AD. *Working memory.* Oxford: Oxford Science Publications, 1986.

Baddeley AD, Hitch GJ. Working memory. In: Bowers G, ed. *Recent advances in learning and motivation.* New York: Academic Press, 1974, 47–90.

Callicott JH, Bertolino A, Mattay VS et al. Physiological dysfunction of the dorsolateral prefrontal cortex in schizophrenia revisited. *Cereb Cortex* 2000; **10**: 1078–92.

Daniel DG, Weinberger DR, Jones DW et al. The effect of amphetamine on regional cerebral blood flow during cognitive activation in schizophrenia. *J Neurosci* 1991; **11**: 1907–17.

Davis KL, Kahn RS, Ko G, Davidson M. Dopamine in schizophrenia: review and re-conceptualization. *Am J Psychiatry* 1991; **148**: 1474–86.

Gold JM, Carpenter C, Randolph C et al. Auditory working memory and the Wisconsin Card Sorting Test in schizophrenia. *Arch Gen Psychiatry* 1997; **54**: 159–65.

Gruzelier J, Seymour K, Wilson L et al. Impairments on neuropsychologic tests of temporohippocampal and frontohippocampal functions and word fluency in remitting schizophrenia and affective disorders. *Arch Gen Psychiatry* 1988; **45**: 623–9.

Harvey PD. Reality monitoring in mania and schizophrenia: the association between thought disorder and performance. *J Nerv Ment Dis* 1985; **173**: 67–73.

Jacobsen CF. Studies of cerebral function in primates. *Comparative Psychology Monographs* 1936; **13**: 1–68.

Johnson MK, Raye CR. Reality monitoring. *Psychol Rev* 1981; **88**: 67–85.

Johnson MK, Hashtroudi S, Lindsay DS. Source monitoring. *Psychol Bull* 1993; **114**: 3–28.

Kahn RS, Harvey PD, Davidson M et al. Neuropsychological correlates of central monoamine function in chronic schizophrenia: relationship between CSF metabolites and cognitive function. *Schizophr Res* 1994; **11**: 217–24.

Keefe RSE. The neurobiology of disturbances of the self: autonoetic agnosia. In: Amador X, David T, eds. *Insight and psychosis.* Oxford: Oxford University Press, 1998.142–73.

Keefe RSE. Working memory dysfunction in schizophrenia. In: Sharma T, Harvey PD, eds. *Cognition in schizophrenia.* Oxford: Oxford University Press, 2000, 16–50.

Okubo Y, Suhara T, Suzuki K et al. Decreased prefrontal dopamine D1 receptors in schizophrenia revealed by PET. *Nature* 1997; **385**: 634–6.

Oscar-Berman M, Bonner RT. Matching- and delayed matching-to-sample performance as measures of visual processing, selective attention, and memory in aging and alcoholic individuals. *Neuropsychologia* 1985; **23**: 639–51.

Sawaguchi T, Goldman-Rakic PS. D1 dopamine receptors in prefrontal cortex: involvement in working memory. *Science* 1991; **251**: 947–50.

Sawaguchi T, Goldman-Rakic PS. The role of D1-dopamine receptor in working memory: local injections of dopamine antagonists into the prefrontal cortex of rhesus. *J Neurophysiol* 1994; **71**: 515–28.

Williams GV, Goldman-Rakic PS. Modulation of memory fields by dopamine DI receptors in prefrontal cortex. *Nature* 1995; **376**: 572–5.

Wilson FAO, O'Scalhaide SP, Goldman-Rakic PS. Dissociation of object and spatial processing domains in primate frontal cortex. *Science* 1993; **260**: 1955–8.

Executive functioning in schizophrenia

5

Executive functioning, as briefly described in Chapter 4 refers to the ability to solve problems, use abstract concepts, and co-ordinate and manage cognitive skills and resources. As result, executive functions are a diverse collection of cognitive abilities and this has led to some confusion and controversy regarding the exact cognitive functions that are executive in nature. Specifically, some researchers believe that working memory is an intrinsically executive function, while others regard executive functions as often dependent upon working memory, but as a discriminable scientific construct. Finally, others see executive functioning as clearly distinct from working memory and believe that the expansion of the concept of working memory to contain the 'central executive' system leads to a conceptual blurring and reduction of focus.

What are the domains of executive functioning?

Like all of the cognitive functioning concepts in the study of schizophrenia, it is possible to separate the theoretical formulation of the concept involved from the specific behavioral tasks used to measure it. Executive functioning clearly includes the ability to solve problems, including formulation of strategies, evaluation of their usefulness, selection of the best strategy, avoiding the effects of irrelevant information, and discarding strategies when they lose their usefulness. Executive functioning also refers to the ability to effectively alternate between competing demands and adaptively shift effort in so doing. Also included in the domains of executive functioning are the ability to manage separate cognitive skills and resources, managing effort without deploying too little to solve a problem or so much as to compromise other ongoing activities.

Other domains that are often referred to as 'executive' include certain verbal skills tasks. In particular, verbal fluency, the ability to produce verbal output based on either semantic or phonological requirements, is often referred to as an executive function. Since these tasks do require a high degree of organization as well as controlled search of lexical storage systems, it is probably appropriate to consider these tasks as indicators of executive functioning.

Is executive functioning the same as 'frontal lobe functioning'?

Lesions to the frontal lobe interfere with many of the cognitive functions just described. Performing tasks that measure these functions activates the frontal lobes in neuroimaging studies (see Chapter 10 for more detail about this). As a result, there is converging evidence that adequate performance of tests of executive functions is dependent on the intactness of the frontal lobes. In the past, these types of functions were often referred to as 'frontal lobe functions'. However, there are reasons to believe that executive functioning and frontal lobe functioning are not exactly the same. There are some frontal lobe functions that are not executive in nature and there is some evidence that the frontal lobe is not solely responsible for performance on executive functioning tests.

The two main sources of physiological evidence that executive functioning tasks are dependent on the frontal lobe, activation of the frontal lobe during performance of these tests (Callicott et al, 2000), and reduction of performance on executive functioning tests with localized lesions (Stuss and Benson, 1986), also are found with even very simple working memory tasks. Some of these working memory tasks are too simple to require any problem solving or strategic selection and can be performed by rodents who have minimal problem solving skills. In addition, lesions in other parts of the brain also reduce performance on classic tests of executive functioning (Anderson et al, 1991). For example, patients who suffer from subcortical dementias that have no direct lesioning effects on the frontal lobes also have executive functioning deficits. Huntington's disease, a progressive condition associated with degeneration of the head of the caudate nucleus, leads to executive functioning deficits as severe as those seen in schizophrenia (Paulsen et al, 1995). These findings may have important implications for the source of executive functioning deficits in schizophrenia.

Tests of executive functioning

There are a number of different tests of executive functioning, all of which have some of the characteristics described above.

The Wisconsin Card Sorting Test

The prototypical test of executive functioning is the Wisconsin Card Sorting Test (WCST). This test, developed in the late 1940s (Berg, 1948) for use as a measure of conceptual functioning, has been used for over five decades to examine patients with schizophrenia. The WCST involves matching cards, which vary along the dimensions of colour, shape, and number. For instance, a stimulus that consists of a single red triangle could be matched to a card containing a red stimulus, a card with triangles, or a single stimulus of any type. In this test, the subject is required to match cards first on colour, then on shape, and then on number. After ten consecutive correct matches, the matching

concept shifts. Thus, this task requires the adoption of a 'win-stay, lose-shift' strategy. In addition, the subject must be able to recognize the sorting concept, remember it while sorting, remember the result of their last response, and respond to feedback by adjusting strategies. An inability to perform any of these skills would render performing this test difficult to impossible, thus highlighting the multiple cognitive components that are required to perform this test.

Patients with schizophrenia have significant problems on this test and many patients cannot even learn how to perform this test with extensive training (Goldberg et al, 1987; Goldberg and Weinberger, 1994). As described in Chapter 7, deficits in performance on this test have specific functional correlates. There is considerable controversy as to whether the most important subcomponent of cognitive dysfunction is responsible for poor performance on the WCST (Gold et al, 1997). A working memory deficit would render performance of this task difficult, because of the problems recalling feedback from the last response or the current sorting concept. A deficit in the ability to perceive conceptual dimensions (i.e. concrete thinking) would render the subject unable to identify the different potential sorting concept. Impulsivity might lead an individual to change concepts before the task demanded a shift in concepts. Thus, while the

WCST is a test that can identify poor problem solving for a variety of different reasons, it does not identify a specific cognitive deficit.

The categories test

This classical neuropsychological test involves the presentation of a series of stimulus sets to which the subject must respond with a choice of the correct item (Heaton et al, 1991; Reitan and Wolfson, 1995). The stimulus sets reflect a conceptual category and the choice of the matching item has to also be the end-product of this ability as well. The rules are always covert and shift across each of the seven sections of the test. There are 208 items on the test and this test is scored in terms of the total number of errors made by the subject. As would be expected, patients with schizophrenia have considerable difficulty on this test and patients who have particular difficulties with the WCST are typically quite impaired on the Categories test as well. There has been much less research with the Categories test than on the WCST, possibly because of the length of the test.

Verbal fluency examinations

Verbal fluency examinations require subjects to produce words that are consistent with several different conceptual demands. For instance, subjects can be asked to produce words that begin with the same letter: 'Tell me as many words as you can that begin with the letter F', or members of the same conceptual categories, such as animals, fruits, or vegetables. Some verbal fluency tests utilize sequential searches of lexical memory, such as producing supermarket items aisle by aisle 'frozen foods followed by canned goods'. Thus, all of the instructions provided require the subjects to organize a semantic or phonological search and to continue to produce information for a controlled period of time, such as 1 min to 90 s per searched item.

Patients with schizophrenia have considerable verbal fluency impairment. Some have argued that their relative impairment is greater on semantic search items such as animals when compared to phonological searches such as letter fluency (Gourovitch et al, 1996). Studies of the correlates of fluency deficits have indicated that memory deficits are more strongly correlated with deficits in phonological fluency and that deficits in other verbal skills, such as confrontation naming, are associated with deficits in category fluency (Harvey et al, 1997). These data are consistent with some research on brain damaged patients suggesting that variations in regional brain damage has different effects on fluency performance.

The Stroop colour word test

The Stroop effect has a long history in experimental psychology and was initially identified in healthy individuals. This test, which has several variants, examines interference effects between semantic concepts, focusing on colours. In the test an individual is asked, in sequence, to read the names of colours (i.e. red, blue) written in black ink, followed by naming the colour of either neutral words or strings of Xs written in coloured inks, followed by naming the colour of the ink in which the names of colours are printed. This final condition is the one that tends to produce the interference effects, where both response latency and error rates increase. Patients with schizophrenia have even more difficulty with this task than healthy individuals, with increases in latency and error rates.

This last finding highlights the diversity of the concept of executive functioning. Performance on the WCST and the Categories test is often completely unimpaired in healthy individuals and the poor performance of patients with schizophrenia is thus an outlying phenomenon. For the Stroop test, performance deficits reflect an exaggeration of a process (i.e. colour response interference) found in healthy individuals. Perhaps this is the reason that there has been considerable controversy regarding the importance of the Stroop test in schizophrenia, with much more difference of opinion regarding the usefulness of this test in neuropsychological assessment than, say, the WCST. In addition, the wide diversity of

methods employed and dependent measures collected reduces the ability of generalizing the findings across different studies of patients with schizophrenia.

Tower tests

There are many different Tower tests employed in schizophrenia research, with the main conceptual similarity being that individuals are asked to plan a series of movements within a set of restrictions, in order to achieve a goal of moving items from one location to another. There are three main versions of the Tower test (see Lezak, 1995): London, Hanoi, and Toronto. In each, the main goal is to move a set of three or four items from one peg to another. In the London test, the restriction is the number of items that can be placed on each of the three pegs, ranging from 1 on the far right to 3 on the left, which is the starting point. In the Hanoi test, the items vary in size and a larger item cannot be placed on a smaller one. Finally, in the Toronto test, the variation is in colour. Typically, the dependent variable is the total number of moves, where effective advance planning rather than trial and error manipulation would reduce the total number of moves executed. A further refinement is that of versions of the test where there is no movement of the items, in that the subject is shown different arrays of items at a hypothetical time point before and after format and asked how many moves it took to get from point A to point B. This version reduces the possibility of increases in scores associated with simple difficulties in physical manipulation of the items and could reflect a purer measure of planning.

Patients with schizophrenia have notable deficits in the Tower tests. Regardless of the version of the test employed, patients make more moves and are more likely to fail to reach any type of criterion regarding trials to completion. One of the problems in this research area is that although these tests seem quite similar, they are found to be poorly correlated with each other. One study found a correlation of only r = 0.37 between these tests, indicating that only 10% of the variance was in common in these seemingly similar tests (Humes et al, 1997). Again highlighting the diversity of the executive functioning concept, even tests that seem very similar may be tapping quite different cognitive processes.

Trail-making test, parts A and B

This test, part of the original Halstead–Reitan Neuropsychological Battery (Reitan and Wolfson, 1995), examines both psychomotor speed and the ability to sustain flexibility while working under time constraints. In part A, the subject simply connects an ascending series of numbers from 1 to 25, presented inside small circles distributed around an 8.5 × 11 (in) sheet. For part B, the subject is instructed to alternate between numbers and letters, connecting 1 to A, then going to 2 and then to B, and so on. Thus, part A measures psychomotor speed under conceptually simple demands, while part B measures the ability to alternate between two different sets of simultaneous demands. Patients with schizophrenia are slower than healthy individuals on both components of this test (Braff et al, 1991). There is some suggestion that they are even slower on Part B, although this is not entirely clear. Thus, before interpreting the performance deficit of a patient with schizophrenia on trail-making part B as reflecting an executive deficit, it is critical to understand their performance on part A.

The overall importance of executive skills deficits in schizophrenia
Everyday functioning

Neurological patients who suffer brain damage and consequential executive functioning deficits manifest disproportionate disability relative to their measured level of intelligence. The classic finding in frontal lobe patients is that their ability to function adaptively is markedly impaired, while a superficial conversation or mental status examination fails to reveal the significance of the impairment (Stuss and Benson, 1986).

While, as noted above, frontal lobe and executive functioning are not identical, there are many similarities. Patients with schizophrenia vary in their executive functioning performance and those who are more impaired have several important clinical features (Green, 1996). They have levels of functional disability that are markedly greater than would be expected on the basis of their IQ. Their impairments in functioning are much greater than would be expected from simple mental status examinations. This functional impairment will be discussed in Chapter 7 in more detail.

Lack of insight

Another correlate of executive functioning deficits can be identified in terms of current symptom status. There are many studies indicating that patients with severe executive functioning deficits are more likely to manifest lack of insight or unawareness of illness. Unawareness of illness refers to the fact that patients with schizophrenia do not recognize symptoms such as delusions or hallucinations as being unusual and not a part of normal experience (Amador et al, 1991). Unawareness of illness is itself correlated with poor medication compliance, self-injurious behavior, and also with risk of violence directed towards others. Several studies have suggested that unawareness of illness may be specifically linked with executive impairments

and not with other cognitive deficits such as attentional or memory impairments (e.g. Young et al, 1993). As a consequence, executive functioning deficits may be associated with several risk factors for poor outcome, including failure to comply with treatment recommendations and dangerousness.

Deficit syndrome and negative symptoms

While negative symptoms have been known to be associated with schizophrenia for decades, the concept of the deficit syndrome is a newer one. The deficit syndrome is defined as a condition where patients, even when in remission from their positive symptoms, have significant negative symptoms, social deficits, and affective impairments (Carpenter et al, 1988). Several different studies have reported that some components of executive functioning are associated with the presence of the deficit syndrome (Buchanan et al, 1994). In fact, executive functioning deficits may be a central feature of this syndrome, which is marked by clear deficits in the ability to engage in motivated and purposeful behavior despite the absence of clear positive symptoms of the illness.

Executive functions and vulnerability to schizophrenia

One of the very interesting features of executive impairments in schizophrenia is that, in contrast to deficits in attention and memory, executive functioning does not appear to be markedly impaired during the prepsychotic period for people who are at risk to develop schizophrenia. This may suggest that part of the early phase of development of schizophrenia may include the development of executive functioning impairment. This is particularly interesting in the context of recent research that suggested that patients who have developed schizophrenia in the absence of generalized intellectual impairments still have evidence of deficits in executive functioning. Thus, executive deficits are often present as the only notable cognitive impairment in patients with only modest evidence of additional cognitive impairments. One of the upcoming challenges will be to identify the brain substrates of these cognitive impairments, which may have many functional and clinical implications. Neuroimaging research presented in Chapter 10 suggests that executive functioning deficits have brain functioning correlates that can be detected.

Conclusions

Executive functioning deficits in schizophrenia are wide-ranging and have multiple clinical and functional correlates. The concept of executive functioning has been somewhat loosely defined and there are often only modest correlations between different tasks that purport to measure executive functions. Furthermore, there is only modest evidence that some tests are measuring cognitive processes that are distinguishable from simpler concepts such as motor speed. It is clear, however, that patients with schizophrenia who have clear evidence of performance deficits on tests such as the WCST have major functional deficits. Although executive functions may be less severely impaired on average than tests of declarative memory (see Chapter 4), executive functioning deficits may be more ubiquitous than memory deficits. This conclusion can be reached from studies showing that patients with schizophrenia with little evidence of major cognitive deficits are still often quite impaired in their ability to perform executive functioning assessments.

The course of executive deficits and their neural substrates are not yet fully understood. The brain substrates of these deficits, and others, will be explored in Chapter 10. In a sense, however, executive skills deficit is the contemporary conceptualization of the 'loss of abstract attitude', a concept that has been embraced as central to the understanding of schizophrenia since it was introduced over 65 years ago. Whether these deficits are referred to as 'concreteness', 'abstraction deficits', 'conceptual overinclusion or conceptual underinclusion', or as executive skills deficits, they reflect a major and important aspect of cognitive impairment in schizophrenia.

References

Amador XF, Strauss DH, Yale SA, Gorman J. Awareness of illness in schizophrenia. *Schizophr Bull* 1991; **17**: 113–32.

Anderson SW, Damasio H, Jones RD, Tranel D. Wisconsin Card Sorting test performance as a measure of frontal lobe damage. *J Clin Exp Neuropsychol* 1991; **13**: 909–22.

Berg EA. Sample objective test for measuring flexibility in thinking. *J Gen Psychol* 1948; **39**: 15–22.

Braff DL, Heaton RK, Kuck J et al. The generalized pattern of neuropsychological deficits in patients with heterogenous WCST results. *Arch Gen Psychiatry* 1991; **48**: 891–8.

Buchanan RW, Strauss ME, Kirkpatrick B et al. Neuropsychological impairments in deficits vs. nondeficit forms of schizophrenia. *Arch Gen Psychiatry* 1994, **51**: 804–11.

Callicott JH, Bertolino A, Mattay VS et al. Physiological dysfunction of the dorsolateral prefrontal cortex in schizophrenia revisited. *Cereb Cortex* 2000; **10**: 1078–92.

Carpenter WT Jr, Heinrichs DW, Wagman AMI. Deficit and nondeficit forms of schizophrenia: the concept. *Am J Psychiatry* 1988; **145**: 578–83.

Gold JM, Carpenter C, Randolph C et al. Auditory working memory and Wisconsin Card Sorting Test performance in schizophrenia. *Arch Gen Psychiatry* 1997; **54**: 159–68.

Goldberg TE, Weinberger DR. Schizophrenia, training paradigms, and the Wisconsin Card Sorting Test redux. *Schizophr Res* 1994; **11**: 291–6.

Goldberg TE, Weinberger DR, Berman KF et al. Further evidence for dementia of the prefrontal type in schizophrenia? A controlled study of teaching the Wisconsin Card Sorting test. *Arch Gen Psychiatry* 1987; **44**: 1008–14.

Gourovitch ML, Goldberg TE, Weinberger DR. Verbal fluency deficits in patients with schizophrenia: semantic fluency is differentially impaired as compared to phonological fluency. *Neuropsychology* 1996; **10**: 573–7.

Green MF. What are the functional consequences of neurocognitive deficits in schizophrenia? *Am J Psychiatry* 1996; **153**: 321–30.

Harvey PD, Leibman M, Lombardi J et al. Verbal fluency in geriatric and nongeriatric chronic schizophrenic patients. *J Neuropsychiatry Clin Neurosci* 1997; **9**: 584–90.

Heaton RK, Grant I, Matthews CG. *Comprehensive norms for an expanded Halstead–Reitan Neuropsychology battery.* Odessa, FL, USA: Psychological Assessment Resources, 1991.

Humes GE, Welsh MC, Retzlaff P, Cookson M. Towers of Hanoi and London: reliability of two executive functioning tests. *Assessment* 1997; **4**: 249–57.

Lezak MD. *Neuropsychological assessment* 3rd edn. Oxford University Press, New York, 1995.

Reitan RM, Wolfson D. Category test and trail making test as measures of frontal lobe functions. *Clin Neuropsychologist* 1995; **9**: 50–6.

Paulsen JS, Butters N, Sadek JR et al. Distinct cognitive profiles of cortical and subcortical dementia in advanced illness. *Neurology* 1995; **45**: 951–6.

Stuss DT, Benson DF. *The frontal lobes.* New York: Raven Press, 1986.

Young DA, Davila R, Scher H. Unawareness of illness and neuropsychological performance in schizophrenia. *Schizophr Res* 1993; **10:** 117–24.

Attention deficits in schizophrenia

6

Among the first cognitive deficits described in schizophrenia were attentional impairments. Kraepelin (1919) and Bleuler (1911) both noted that patients with schizophrenia had difficulties in attentional focus. These attentional focus deficits include both the ability to sustain attention on appropriate stimuli and the ability to attend selectively to relevant as compared to irrelevant aspects of the stimulus situation. Since the early days of schizophrenia research, conceptualizations of attentional functioning have become more sophisticated, as have the techniques employed to measure them. This chapter will examine attention in schizophrenia, possibly one of the most important aspects of cognitive deficit in the illness.

The components of attentional functioning

Attention refers to the set of operations that enable the individual to identify relevant stimuli in the environment (detection), focus on that stimulus rather than others (selective attention), sustain focus on the stimulus until it is processed (sustained attention), and allow for transfer of the stimulus to higher-level processes. Thus, the cognitive processes at the boundaries between perception and memory are those that are designated as attentional functions, with these distinctions being always somewhat arbitrary.

Directional processing

Processing of environmental stimuli can occur in either a 'bottom-up' or a 'top-down' manner. Bottom-up processing is stimulus driven, in that stimuli that impinge on perceptual processing are then processed 'up the line'. This means that stimuli that are detected are focused on, kept in attention, analysed, and then processed more deeply if they are determined by higher level cognitive functions to be relevant to the current situation. Top-down processing refers to processing of information that is intentionally sought out in the environment and then processed in the same general sequence. For instance, familiar stimuli are generally attended to more effectively than completely novel stimuli, meaning that recognition memory processes effectively activate the attentional apparatus. Thus, attentional impairments can theoretically originate from deficits at any stage of the processing stream as well as from the inability to direct attentional functions in order to efficiently identify information in the environment. As a result, executive control over attentional functions is critical, again demonstrating the inter-

relatedness of cognitive processes in both normal cognition and in schizophrenia.

Processing capacity

There are always multiple sources of information in the environment. It is, therefore, adaptively important to perform some aspects of information processing simultaneously; this is referred to as 'parallel processing'. Some information processing tasks can only be performed individually and one task must be completed before the next is initiated, with this process referred to 'serial processing'. For instance, it is easy to talk and walk at the same time, while it is more difficult to talk and to type at the same time and even more difficult to talk and sing at the same time. It is also believed that there is a finite amount of processing resources available at any given time, with this amount of processing capacity varying across individuals and influenced by several different environmental and pharmacological variables.

Some serial processes can become parallel with practice, referred to as the process of 'automating' previously 'controlled' processes. For instance, driving is a process that is initiated in a serial manner and becomes more and more automated with practice. Beginner drivers often cannot talk and drive at the same time and have difficulties simultaneously operating the different controls (i.e. windshield wipers and gearshift) of the automobile while driving. With practice, multiple tasks can be performed while driving, such as operating vehicle controls, listening to the radio, and engaging in conversation. A critical part of normal skill acquisition is the development of automatic processing of these simple, often procedural (see Chapter 3), skills. The more difficult or multifaceted the skill, the more time and practice it takes before it can be performed automatically.

The critical defining characteristic of the level of difficulty or resource demands of a task is the extent to which performance deteriorates when additional processing demands are added. This experimental procedure, referred to as 'dual task processing' or 'divided attentional processing', is used to determine the level of resource demands of different tasks. A task that can be performed equally well with or without another task being added is referred to as being performed in an automated manner. Thus, the level of demand of any single task can be indexed by how much performance on another resource-demanding task declines when that first task is added.

An additional critical feature in dual task processing is assessment of processing strategy. If a subject is instructed to divide attention equally and does not, then one task may deteriorate disproportionately. Thus, assessment of the strategic aspects of information processing allows for the separation of executive functioning problems

(i.e. misallocation of resources) from processing capacity limitations (i.e. inability to perform despite adequate allocation of effort).

Selective attention

Selective attention or focused attention refers to the ability to train attention on a certain aspect of the environment while ignoring other environmental stimuli. A real-world example would be listening to someone on the telephone tell you their telephone number while you are working in a busy office where there are multiple additional conversations occurring simultaneously in the background. Since there are nearly always potential competing stimuli in any environmental situation, selective attention is a constant process. Selective attention is a critical feature of dual task information processing, because it can be shown that ignoring particularly salient environmental stimuli requires effort and processing resources. Selective attention is often measured with tests that present target stimuli in the presence of irrelevant stimuli, with the relevant and irrelevant information often separable on the basis of some rule (e.g. listen to the woman and ignore all the male voices).

Sustained attention

Sustained attention or vigilance refers to the process of sustaining attention and effort while processing stimuli that are relatively rare in their frequency. A real-world example of this process would be a security guard monitoring several video monitors simultaneously, while most of the monitors are showing nothing most of the time. The classical test of vigilance is the continuous performance test (CPT; Rosvold et al, 1956). In this test, a subject is instructed to watch a series of continuously presented informational stimuli while only making a response to a predetermined stimulus or target sequence. These stimuli can be letters, numbers, or nonsense shapes and can be presented in either the visual or auditory sensory modality. This test can identify both inattention (i.e. failures to respond to targets) or impulsivity (i.e. responses to nontarget stimuli) in the same testing session. There are several different versions of the CPT, which include responses both to predetermined target sequences (e.g. 3–7; Nuechterlein et al, 1986), the same stimulus when it occurs twice in succession (e.g. Cornblatt et al, 1989), or versions where the target stimuli are perceptually degraded (Nuechterlein et al, 1986).

Rapid visual processing

There are several different paradigms that have been used to measure the processing of information that is presented for brief durations. These paradigms include the Span of Apprehension Test (Asarnow et al, 1988) and the visual Backward masking paradigms (Green et al, 1994). In both paradigms a stimulus such as a letter is presented for a very brief period and the subject is asked if the letter was one of two possible letters. For the span of apprehension, the stimulus is presented either alone or in the presence of several irrelevant letters and for the backward masking task the stimulus is presented rapidly and then is covered by a mask of randomly distributed visual 'noise' stimulation. Both of these tasks assess the ability to process information presented for a very brief period, while the span of apprehension has the additional feature of examining the effects of irrelevant information.

There are a large number of attentional concepts in schizophrenia that have been measured with relatively standardized tests. The concepts and tests are presented in Table 6.1.

Information processing deficits in schizophrenia

Patients with schizophrenia also show slower rates of development of automatic information processing with practice (Granholm et al, 1991 and 1996a; Serper et al, 1990). These deficits do not include every aspect of information processing in schizophrenia, however. For example, while patients with schizophrenia deteriorate more than healthy individuals when asked to

Table 6.1
Attentional domains and tests

Domain	Test
Selective attention/distractibility	Digit span distraction test
Sustained attention/vigilance	Continuous performance test
Rapid visual processing	Span of apprehension
	Backward masking
Attentional capacity	Dual task/divided attention tests

perform divided attention tests, they appear to utilize normal processing strategies (Granholm et al, 1996a). Specifically, patients with schizophrenia do not manifest abnormalities in the ways that they allocate their attention, inappropriately prioritizing one task over another. This finding suggests that executive control of attentional functions is not the principal cause of impairment in performance on information processing tasks. Similarly, patients with schizophrenia do not identify individual target letters with less accuracy than healthy individuals on the span of apprehension test, suggesting that their performance deficits are related to selective attention processes and not simply due to excessively slow processing.

Clinical correlates of information processing deficits

In contrast to other types of cognitive deficits, attentional deficits appear more strongly linked to symptoms of disorganization, such as formal thought disorder, than to negative symptoms. For instance, patients with schizophrenia who are highly distractible (i.e. have poor selective attention) have higher levels of formal thought disorder (Harvey et al, 1988). Similar findings have been reported for the CPT (Nuechterlein et al, 1986) and other information processing measures (Perry and Braff, 1994). Impairment in performance on other measures of information processing, such as backward masking (Braff, 1989), is associated with the presence of more severe negative symptoms. Thus, attentional deficits may have more of a role than other aspects of cognitive functioning, such as memory or executive functioning deficits, in the genesis of different schizophrenic symptoms.

Psychophysiological correlates of information processing deficits

When patients with schizophrenia perform poorly on attentional tests, indices of physiological reactivity are also impacted. For instance, measures of pupillary diameter, known to track response to information processing load in healthy individuals, suggest that patients with schizophrenia are experiencing cognitive overload conditions at much lower levels of load than healthy individuals. This finding is consistent across both psychophysiological (Granholm et al, 1996b) and attentional tasks (Granholm et al, 1997). Thus, the evidence for processing capacity limitations is greater than that for strategic failures in these attention demanding tasks.

Additional evidence of the psychophysiological substrates of these processing deficits is provided by the results of studies of startle response in schizophrenia. Patients with schizophrenia fail to develop habituation to previously startling stimuli, acting as if each stimulus was novel. An additional finding is that informing or cuing the patient that they are about to be startled does not reduce the extent of their startle response (Braff and Geyer, 1990). In healthy individuals a cue before the occurrence of a previously experienced startling stimulus partially to completely eliminates the startle response, increasingly with repeated exposures. This 'pre-pulse inhibition' phenomenon is reduced markedly in schizophrenia patients and is sometimes completely absent.

The potential implications of these startle abnormalities are quite significant. Absence of normal habituation of startle response would subject an individual to the subjective experience of exposure to high energy stimuli on a regular basis and would also mean that the world in general would be a more threatening and stressful environment. Modulation of the startle response has a variety of adaptive functions and several different theories have suggested how unattenuated startling stimuli could have the potential to lead to both hallucinations, based on the repeated experience of intrusive stimuli, and delusions, based on attempts to explain the high level of sensory overload experienced.

The course of attentional deficits

Similar to most other aspects of cognitive deficit in schizophrenia, attentional impairments appear to persist after remission of acute psychotic episodes. Performance on the CPT and span of apprehension test (Asarnow et al, 1978), susceptibility to distraction (Harvey et al, 1990), and other attentional functions such as pre-pulse inhibition (Cadenhead et al, 1997) is unaffected by the remission of psychotic symptoms. These persistent attentional deficits are not likely to be a consequence of treatment with antipsychotic medications, because, more than other aspects of cognitive deficit in schizophrenia, even conventional medications reduce some of these attentional impairments (Oltmanns et al, 1979; Serper et al, 1994). Furthermore, attentional deficits are also clearly present in unmedicated patients (Harvey and Pedley, 1989) and comparison of patients prior to and after treatment reveals, if anything, shows an attenuation of attentional deficits (Serper et al, 1994).

Attentional deficits as markers of vulnerability

Perhaps more than any other aspect of cognitive functioning, attentional deficits are strong candidates as markers of vulnerability. As described above, attentional deficits have been shown to persist in patients with schizophrenia who were largely in remission of their symptoms. In addition, later studies have shown the potentially important role of these factors as markers of vulnerability to schizophrenia. Children of schizophrenic parents have deficits in both sustained (Asarnow et al, 1977) and selective attention (Harvey et al, 1981), widely replicated across studies. Individuals with schizotypal personality disorder also demonstrate deficits in both sustained attention and rapid visual processing (Braff, 1981; Harvey et al, 1996).

The most compelling data in this regard have been reported by the New York High Risk project, with Drs. L. Erlenmeyer-Kimling and Barbara Cornblatt as the most

consistent and visible contributors. This long-term study has followed a sample of children of schizophrenic parents for periods of up to 30 years. Starting while these children were in the early years of elementary school, they have been followed with repeated assessments of various cognitive, clinical, functional, and personality measures. Their study is unique in that it contained comparison samples of children of psychiatrically ill, nonschizophrenic parents and the children of healthy controls. Instead of focusing in a single aspect of cognitive functioning, the assessment was relatively wide ranging, allowing for interpretation of the specificity of the results.

This study has produced two findings of singular importance. The first was that global attentional deviance, defined as impairments across multiple measures of attentional functioning, was a prime discriminator between children of schizophrenic and nonschizophrenic parents (Cornblatt and Erlenmeyer-Kimling, 1985). Thus, these results suggested that individual domains of attentional functioning were largely nonspecific to schizophrenia, while the presence of multiple deficits identified children of schizophrenic parents. Even more striking, the results of the second study suggested that children followed from around age 12 years until their mid-30s could be separated into those who would develop schizophrenia and related conditions and those who would not, with around 85% specificity (Cornblatt et al, 1999). Simply put, children of schizophrenic parents without global attentional deviance had no higher risk for schizophrenia than the children of normal parents and the children of affectively ill parents. The level of attentional deviance seen in the 12 year olds who later developed schizophrenia was considerable when compared to the comparison samples, but actually worsened slightly at around the time of the first episode. No changes in

performance were seen after the development of the illness, suggesting that the illness itself does not markedly affect performance on this set of measures. Figure 6.1 presents the course of these cognitive attentional deficits, as presented in the latest of these reports.

The data from this study suggest that attentional impairments are potential markers of vulnerability to the development of schizophrenia and that in samples of children of schizophrenic parents, there may be some predictive power. The data also suggest that a

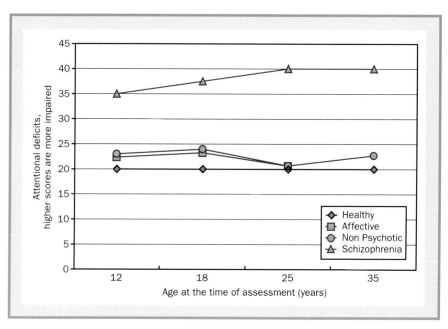

Figure 6.1
Performance of children of psychiatric patients and healthy patients as a function of adult outcome. Adapted from Cornblatt et al, 1999.

single attentional deficit is not likely to have prognostic importance and that an array of measures may be required in order to identify the profile of vulnerability in this population.

The functional importance of attentional deficits

As described in the next chapter, the functional importance of deficits in attention and information processing is considerable. Clearly this makes conceptual sense. If it is impossible to identify and focus on information in the environment, then social information processing, educational, and occupational attainment will necessarily be limited. Regardless of whether attention and information processing are the most important predictors of functional status, their relationship with functional deficits seems extremely easy to understand. As important is the notion that patients with schizophrenia fail to inhibit the influence of startling stimuli. It is difficult to estimate the consequences of living in a world where every stimulus is completely novel, and quite possibly startling to the point of being unsettling. The sound of an ambulance passing by in an urban area would have the same impact the 500th time that it happened as the first, and similarly upsetting stimuli that we all eventually adjust to (pictures on the evening news for example) would also fail to lose their shock value over time. As a result, the inability to adjust

physiological reactivity to experience can have a large-scale emotional impact as well as a functional one.

Can attentional deficits be used for primary prevention?

Schizophrenia is a devastating illness that has a major impact across the entire lifespan. Anything that could identify high-risk individuals and then provide an intervention would be a major public health breakthrough. The high level of predictive power in the studies from the New York High Risk Project superficially seems to suggest that large-scale screening for attentional deficits could have a major public health benefit. After all, if one can identify with 85% accuracy by age 12 years the individuals who will develop schizophrenia, a wide array of preventive interventions could be attempted before the major onset of the age of risk 6–20 years later. While it may eventually prove true that attentional deficits can identify individuals at risk for schizophrenia, there are several caveats that must be considered. The sample of the New York High Risk Project was limited to children of schizophrenic parents. This population has a risk for schizophrenia that is 10 to 15 times higher than the general population (although their risk is actually not extremely high when compared to other genetic illnesses such as Huntington's disease). The efficiency of prediction might be reduced in the general population with its much lower base rate of occurrence of the illness. Furthermore, the risk factors for the development of schizophrenia might be different in a population where the genetic predisposing factors are less clear. Thus, attentional deficits might only be a powerful predictor in this type of genetically predisposed high-risk population.

A further complicating factor is the fact that relatives of patients with schizophrenia who are old enough to have passed through the majority of the age of risk also manifest attentional deficits. In studies of older relatives of patients with schizophrenia, deficits in sustained attention are found to correlate with the likelihood of having symptoms of schizotypal personality disorder (Keefe et al, 1997). As a result, attentional deficits must either change dynamically over time, developing in individuals who are not at risk for schizophrenia, or must be associated with a high rate of false positive prediction for development of the illness.

Thus, several factors complicate the use of any type of attentional screening to initiate primary prevention. Independent of the ethical considerations involved (after all, 85% specificity still means 15% false positives even in the high risk samples), there are no data to suggest that schizophrenia in general population samples can be predicted with anything close to the same efficiency as in the high risk samples. For now, the data suggest

that populations of younger individuals who are related to individuals with schizophrenia could potentially be considered for these programs, if they can be identified in the first place. Such programs would necessarily be limited to urban or large-scale rural catchment areas and these findings of high predictive specificity, because of their unique nature, have not yet or may never be replicated.

Conclusion

Deficits in attention and information processing are widely present in patients with schizophrenia and occur over the entire course of the illness. These deficits are present before, during, and after psychotic episodes. Patients with schizophrenia have a wide array of attentional deficits, but are not impaired on all aspects of information processing. In particular, information processing deficits are not due to strategic failures or to simple reductions in processing speed. These attentional deficits have measurable psychophysiological correlates and patients with schizophrenia show reductions in their ability to adapt to prior experience, in the domains of habituation of startle responses and developing automatic processing skills.

Attentional impairments are probably the most promising candidates for markers of vulnerability to schizophrenia. In particular, children of parents with schizophrenia who go on to develop schizophrenia have notable deficits in attentional functioning that are detectable far in advance of any other symptoms of the illness. At the same time, primary prevention efforts are not necessarily indicated yet, because of the lack of information about the predictor profile of vulnerability processes in individuals who do not have a first degree relative with schizophrenia.

References

Asarnow RF, MacCrimmon D. Residual performance deficit in clinically remitted schizophrenics: a marker of schizophrenia? *J Abnorm Psychol* 1978; **87**: 597–608.

Asarnow RF, Marder SR, Mintz J et al. Differential effect of low and conventional doses of fluphenazine on schizophrenic outpatients with good and poor information-processing abilities. *Arch Gen Psychiatry* 1988; **45**: 822–6.

Asarnow RF, Steffy R, Cleghorn JM, MacCrimmon DJ. Attentional assessment of foster children vulnerable to schizophrenia. *J Abnorm Psychol* 1977; **86**: 267–75.

Bleuler, E. *Dementia praecox; or the group of schizophrenias.* New York: International Universities Press, 1911.

Braff DL. Impaired speed of information processing in unmedicated schizotypal patients *Schizophr Bull* 1981; 7: 499–508.

Braff DL. Sensory input deficits and negative symptoms in schizophrenic patients. *Am J Psychiatry* 1989; **146**: 1006–11.

Braff DL, Geyer MA. Sensorimotor gating and schizophrenia: human and animal studies. *Arch Gen Psychiatry* 1990; **47**: 181–8.

Cadenhead KS, Geyer MA, Butler RW et al. Information processing deficits of schizophrenic patients: relationship to clinical ratings, gender, and medication status. *Schizophr Res* 1997; **28**: 51–62.

Cornblatt BA, Erlenmeyer-Kimling L. Global attentional deviance as a marker of risk for schizophrenia: Specificity and predictive validity. *J Abnorm Psychol* 1985; **94**: 470–86.

Cornblatt BA, Lenzenweger MF, Erlenmeyer-Kimling L. The continuous performance test, identical pairs version. II. Contrasting attentional profiles in schizophrenic and depressed patients. *Psychiatry Res* 1989; **29**: 65–85.

Cornblatt B, Obuchowski M, Roberts S, Erlenmeyer-Kimling L. Cognitive and behavioral precursors of schizophrenia. *Dev Psychopathol* 1999; **11**: 487–508.

Granholm E., Asarnow RF, Marder S. Controlled information resources and the development of automatic detection responses in schizophrenia. *J Abnorm Psychol* 1991; **100**: 22–30.

Granholm E., Asarnow RF, Marder SR. Dual task performance operating characteristics, resource limitations, and automatic processing in schizophrenia. *Neuropsychology* 1996a; **10**: 3–11.

Granholm E, Asarnow RF, Sarkin AJ, Dykes KL. Pupillary responses index resource limitations. *Psychophysiology* 1996b; **33**: 457–61.

Granholm E, Morris SK, Sarkin AJ et al. Pupillary responses index overload of working memory resources in schizophrenia. *J Abnorm Psychol* 1997; **106**: 458–67.

Green MF, Nuechterlein KH, Mintz J. Backward masking in schizophrenia and mania. I. Specifying a mechanism. *Arch Gen Psychiatry* 1994; **51**: 939–44.

Harvey PD, Docherty N, Serper MR, Rasmussen M. Cognitive deficits and thought disorder: II.

An eight-month follow-up study. *Schizophr Bull* 1990; **16**: 147–56.

Harvey PD, Earle-Boyer EA, Levinson JC. Cognitive deficits and thought disorder: a retest study. *Schizophr Bull* 1988; **14**: 57–66.

Harvey PD, Mohs RC, Keefe RSE et al. Information processing markers of vulnerability to schizophrenia: performance of patients with schizotypal and nonschizotypal personality disorders. *Psychiatry Res* 1996; **60**: 49–56.

Harvey PD, Pedley M. Auditory and visual distractibility in schizophrenics: clinical and medication status correlations. *Schizophr Res* 1989; **2**: 295–300.

Harvey P, Winters K, Weintraub S, Neale JM. Distractibility in children vulnerable to psychopathology. *J Abnorm Psychol* 1981; **90**: 298–304.

Keefe RSE, Silverman JM, Mohs RC et al. Eye-tracking, attention, and schizotypal personality symptoms in nonpsychotic relatives of schizophrenic patients. *Arch Gen Psychiatry* 1997; **54**: 169–77.

Kraepelin E. *Dementia praecox and paraphrenia.* Edinburgh: E & S Livingstone, 1919.

Nuechterlein KH, Edell WS, Norris M, Dawson ME. Attentional vulnerability indicators, thought disorder, and negative symptoms. *Schizophr Bull* 1986; **12**: 408–26.

Oltmanns TF, Ohayon J, Neale JM. The effect of medication and diagnostic criteria on distractibility in schizophrenia. *J Psychiatric Res* 1979; **14**: 81–91.

Perry W, Braff DL. Information-processing deficits and thought disorder in schizophrenia. *Am J Psychiatry* 1994; **151**: 363–7.

Rosvold HE, Mirsky A, Sarason L et al. A continuous performance test of brain damage. *J Consult Psychology* 1956; **20**: 34–50.

Serper MR, Bergman RL, Harvey PD. Medication may be required for the development of automatic information processing in schizophrenia. *Psychiatry Res* 1990; **32**: 281–8.

Serper MR, Davidson M, Harvey PD. Attentional predictors of clinical change during neuroleptic treatment. *Schizophr Res* 1994; **13**: 65–71.

Functional deficits and cognition

7

Functional impairments in schizophrenia

There is only one symptom of schizophrenia that is present, by definition, in every patient. A diagnosis of schizophrenia can be made according to DSM or ICD criteria if a patient has never had a delusion or a hallucination, because the combined presence of two or more other features of schizophrenia, including negative symptoms, communication impairments, or bizarre behavior are sufficient to substantiate the diagnosis of schizophrenia. However, a decline in functioning that has persisted for at least 6 months is required for the schizophrenia diagnosis. Thus, much like cognitive deficits, functional deficits are present in most patients and the level of impairment is quite substantial.

There are several different dimensions of functional deficit in schizophrenia. Patients with schizophrenia have marked impairments in independent living, social functioning, occupational skills, and self-care. The level of severity of these impairments is also quite substantial. For example, most patients with schizophrenia require some sort of public funding for their support and this pattern of dependence develops early in the illness. As many as 50% of first episode patients with schizophrenia are receiving a disability allowance within the first 6 months of their illness (Ho et al, 1997). Social functioning deficits are manifested by the reduced reproductive efficiency of patients with schizophrenia, particularly males. Fewer than 10% of all male patients with schizophrenia ever have a child, highlighting the deficits in initiation and maintenance of social functioning seen in the illness. Occupational functioning is grossly impaired, with as few as 10% of patients with schizophrenia working full time in competitive employment and only 20% of patients able to sustain supported employment on a part-time basis. Finally, self-care deficits are reflected in substantial medical co-morbidity, especially in outpatients with schizophrenia. Patients with schizophrenia typically last as little as 6 months when referred to a job and a surprising number are only employed for a single day.

The course of functional deficits in schizophrenia

Functioning before the onset of schizophrenia, referred to as premorbid adjustment, has been known for years to predict the course of functional outcome in schizophrenia (Langfelt, 1937). Patients with relatively poorer social, academic, occupational, and independent living capacity before the formal diagnosis of the illness have been found to be more likely to have poorer adjustment during the illness. Functional impairments after the onset are predicted by lower premorbid educational attainment (Swanson et al, 1998), poorer premorbid scholastic performance (Wieselgren and Lindstrom, 1996), impaired premorbid socio-sexual functioning (Keefe et al, 1989), and premorbid failure to live independently (Bailer et al, 1996). In addition, patients with relatively earlier ages of onset have been found to typically have poorer adjustment as well (Johnstone et al, 1989), including poorer response to antipsychotic treatment (Meltzer et al, 1997). Thus, functional impairment prior to the onset of the illness predicts functional status during the illness. This should be no surprise, because a patient who has never had an independent residence, a stable job, and social functioning before they experienced psychotic symptoms would hardly be expected to suddenly develop those skills for the first time after the onset of serious psychotic illness.

During the course of the illness most patients experience stable functional impairments, with little evidence of full recovery on the part of most patients. Full recovery is reported in about 10–20% of patients with schizophrenia and functional deterioration before the geriatric years occurs in a smaller portion of these patients. Some patients develop a poor outcome syndrome where they become completely dependent on others for all of their care over the course of their life (Keefe et al, 1987). It is not clear what proportion of patients with schizophrenia become persistently dysfunctional in this manner, but it appears likely that about 10–20% of patients with schizophrenia remain completely and persistently disabled, often requiring institutional care or other high-service, continuous interventions. In contrast to the episodic course of psychotic symptoms, functional impairments tend to be quite stable over time in all patients and not just in those with severely impaired outcome.

Treatment of functional deficits

Functional impairments have typically been treated with behavioral interventions aimed at skills training. These interventions have typically attempted to teach social, occupational, self-care, and independent living skills through a variety of behavioral techniques. Such training programs have employed a variety of strategies, including reinforcement contingencies (such as token economies), social skills training, supported employment, and cognitive-behavioral therapies. Shared among these interventions is a model that the patients need to acquire and deploy new skills and strategies, in a structured and step-by-step model.

The level of success of these interventions has been relatively limited, when compared to the results of pharmacological interventions aimed at the reduction of psychotic symptoms. For instance, even with conventional antipsychotic treatment, only 25% of patients with schizophrenia manifest persistent psychotic symptoms (Lieberman, 1999) and at the time of the first episode, as many as 90% of patients respond to treatment with a remission of their psychotic symptoms (Robinson et al, 1999). In contrast, despite the variety of behavioral interventions applied to patients with schizophrenia for over 10 decades, the overall level of outcome has not been markedly improved (Hegarty et al, 1994). This finding indicates that some other factor may be intervening to reduce the effectiveness of these interventions.

Cognition and outcome

Since the early 1970s it has been recognized that cognitive impairments are the primary factor affecting outcome from a variety of neurological and neuropsychiatric conditions (Heaton and Pendleton 1981). This finding makes logical sense, in that for most neurological conditions functional impairments occur only after the occurrence of events that compromise cognitive functioning. In progressive conditions such as Alzheimer's disease and Huntington's disease, functional impairments follow the course of cognitive changes (Stern et al, 1994). For instance, inability to perform occupational activities or home responsibilities occurs later in the course of the illness of Alzheimer's disease, not at the very outset. Progression of the illness is typically conceptualized in terms of the joint progression of cognitive and functional impairments.

Studies of global outcome in patients with schizophrenia have revealed relationships between overall outcome, defined in terms of chronic institutionalization versus lifelong ambulatory status, and cognitive functioning. In particular, chronically institutionalized patients have more severe cognitive deficits than patients with a lifelong history of occasional relatively brief psychotic episodes (Perlick et al, 1992), even if the better-outcome patients are assessed while experiencing a psychotic episode (Harvey et al, 1998). In addition, patients with more severe cognitive deficits at the time of their first episode are more likely to develop a chronic course of illness (Breier et al, 1991), being more likely to develop a pattern of treatment nonresponse, to be unemployed, and to fail to live independently.

Cognition and outcome: specific correlations

Patients with schizophrenia are found to manifest a specific pattern of relationships between cognitive deficits and specific functional limitations (see Green 1996 and

Green et al, 2000a for detailed descriptions). Not all of the domains of cognitive deficit in schizophrenia are found to relate to functional status, with only a limited set of cognitive deficits found to consistently predict functional limitations. Interestingly, the domain of cognitive functioning in schizophrenia that has consistently shown itself to be unrelated to functional outcome is verbal IQ scores. In contrast, in western cultures in general, verbal skills, particularly IQ, are potent predictors of functional outcome. For each of the multiple domains of functional deficit, specific cognitive impairments have been shown to predict the severity of impairment. Table 7.1 shows the important domains of cognitive deficit in schizophrenia and the aspects of functional impairment with which they have been shown previously to be correlated. As can be seen in this table, each of these functional domains has an array of different cognitive deficits that are related to impairments in that skills area. The most consistent correlate of functional outcome across domains is declarative memory. Perhaps this should not be surprising. Social, occupational, and independent living tasks require the ability to learn new information and to use that information in an adaptive manner. In social situations, if one cannot learn the names of new acquaintances it would be very difficult to engage them in conversation or to develop relationships.

Table 7.1
Functional impairments and their cognitive correlates

Functional domain	Cognitive correlates
Social functions	Declarative memory Vigilance
Occupational functioning	Executive functions Declarative memory Working memory Vigilance
Independent living	Executive functions Declarative memory Working memory

Occupationally, if one is unable to learn the skills that are required to perform work-related tasks, then skills would never be perfected. Even seemingly unskilled labour often has high levels of memory demands. For instance, if the job that you are required to do is digging a hole, there is often the demand that the dirt be thrown on the correct side of the excavation site. Likewise, in a rapidly advancing technological society, what constitutes unskilled employment often changes rapidly. At this time, data entry is viewed as unskilled labour, as is working at a cash register using a complex touch-screen routine to check out sales. Clearly these jobs have a high level of learning demands, demands that are far beyond the capacity of an individual whose memory performance is at the 1st percentile of the normal

distribution. Finally, independent living poses a number of memory challenges. The challenges range from the basic (recalling one's address and the route from home to different appointments; paying the rent on the first of the month) to the complex, such as recalling the contents of a list of items to be purchased to stock the pantry and keep the home supplied.

Executive functioning is also clearly implicated in a number of occupational and independent living tasks. In the occupational domain, many seemingly unskilled tasks have high levels of executive demands. Working in a full-service fuel station requires the execution of at least eight discrete steps in exact order many times per hour. While each of the steps is both cognitively and behaviourally simple, the order is critical. None of these steps can be omitted or performed out of sequence. Planning for the future is a regular feature of independent living, from the seemingly trivial task of ensuring that there is milk for the coffee in the morning to the more complex issues of financial planning and saving for the future. Working memory appears intrinsically linked to many of these functional domains as well. In order to proceed through a series of occupational or home-related tasks it is important to be able to remember which tasks are completed and which are yet to be initiated. As presented in Chapter 5, the intrinsic working memory demands of different executive functioning tasks suggest that these two domains are highly related in areas regarding sequences of activities that are required to maintain the residence.

The finding that vigilance is consistently associated with social skills deficits is the only area where the relationship does not have a common-sense relationship. It may be that maintenance of a consistent cognitive and attentional focus is a key aspect of smooth interpersonal interactions. Providing the appearance of paying attention is crucial in order to have the listener conclude that you are interested in what they are saying, while the overt appearance of not attending may be perceived as reflecting lack of interest or even rudeness. It may also be that vigilance reflects some initial stage in the ability to initiate personal interactions. The ability to focus on subtle interpersonal cues and sustain focus on the listener's affective and verbal reactions to your communication is likely to allow interactions to get off to a good start as well. Without the ability to remain engaged in an interaction, the interaction will falter and seem strained to all of the parties involved.

Cognition and rehabilitation: possible interference effects

A number of studies have examined the relationship between cognitive functioning and progress in rehabilitation. Similar to employment, rehabilitation is also a situation where there are substantial cognitive demands placed on the patients. After all, psychiatric rehabilitation is based on learning models and most of these treatments have a curriculum, structured learning experiences, and what amounts to constant testing of the patient (Bellack et al, 1997). Perhaps it is no surprise that individuals who have significant deficits in their ability to learn information, including information as basic as simple attentional skills, have a reduced rate of learning when exposed to the teaching of complex social and interpersonal skills. Several studies have suggested that patients with schizophrenia whose memory skills (Mueser et al, 1991) and vigilance performance (Bowen et al, 1994; Kern et al, 1992) are the poorest are also the patients who profit the least from social skills training. Thus, cognitive impairments are predictors of functional deficits at baseline and also may be 'rate-limiters' as far as the acquisition of skills when patients are exposed to training.

Several studies have suggested that, despite their seeming importance for interfering with rehabilitation, positive, negative, and disorganized symptoms of schizophrenia do not correlate with progress in rehabilitation (Mueser et al, 1997). While some patients whose symptoms are extremely severe are not likely to be referred to rehabilitation, especially if they are violent or disruptive, the range of symptom severity of patients receiving rehabilitation treatments is quite wide. As a result, symptom factors appear less salient than cognitive factors when predicting rehabilitation success (Velligan et al, 1997). Some studies have suggested that both cognitive deficits and negative symptoms independently predict reductions in benefit from rehabilitation interventions (Breier et al, 1991). It is clear, however, that negative symptoms are much more predictive than the other two major symptom dimensions of rehabilitation success. In addition, no studies that have examined both cognitive and negative symptoms have found that negative symptoms were better predictors of rehabilitation failures than cognitive deficits.

The reason for the lack of relationship of positive and disorganized symptoms and rehabilitation outcome is similar to the reason for the lack of relationship between cognitive deficits and these symptoms. These two domains of symptoms are cyclical and responsive, in most patients, to treatment with antipsychotic medications. Many patients who fail in rehabilitation have essentially no positive symptoms, but they have marked deficits in their cognitive functioning.

One of the important factors to keep in mind when considering rates of learning with training is which types of patients are referred to rehabilitation. The most common candidate for rehabilitation treatment is a patient with a long history of chronic hospitalization, extensive functional deficit, and other associated impairments. As noted above, these are the patients who are likely to have most severe cognitive impairments and to have impairments in the greatest number of the cognitive domains that are linked to functional outcome. Thus, a subsample of patients with schizophrenia who are least likely to be able to attend to, focus on, and learn new information are selected for intensive learning interventions. These patients then show fairly slow rates of learning and receive only modest benefit from rehabilitation. Needless to say, the frustration experienced by someone who is placed in a situation where they simply do not have the skills to perform is likely to make them drop out. For some of these patients, the discrepancy between their skills and the demands of psychiatric rehabilitation is consistent with asking a beginner football player to play for a first division team.

In contrast, in current acute care settings, individuals who are relatively high functioning, for patients with schizophrenia, are often not referred to rehabilitation settings. For instance, a college undergraduate who experiences a psychotic episode often receives the advice to return to college after the remission of symptoms. As noted in Chapter 2, just because an individual has a history of high levels of cognitive functioning there is no guarantee that they have not experienced a deterioration in their cognitive functioning associated with the onset of schizophrenia. Such an individual is quite likely to be functioning more poorly in one or more cognitive domains than before the onset of schizophrenia, with the result being that when they attempt to return to college they fail their courses and drop out.

Our suggestion is that cognitive functioning should be considered at the time of assignment to rehabilitation interventions (Mueser, 2000). Among the patients who are most likely to benefit from rehabilitation are the patients who we often see as not in need of this type of intervention. These include patients with higher levels of premorbid cognitive functioning and those patients early in the course of illness. Among the patients least likely to benefit, at least at present, are the patients typically sent to rehabilitation. These are patients with a chronic course of illness, poor premorbid functioning, no history of occupational or social success at any level, and grossly impaired cognitive functions. In other areas of medicine, triage is considered to be a reasonable strategy, where patients who have the most urgent needs or those who are likely to receive benefit are treated first. In psychiatric rehabilitation, patients who are most likely to receive benefit should be treated first. Patients who stay in rehabilitation programs for 5 to 10 years are, by any reasonable definition of functional outcome, not a success. Yet, these are all too often the typical patients in these programs. Patients who are treated for a year or less and who can succeed in employment and independent living are the successes in rehabilitation. The patient who is most likely to achieve rapid success is the patient whose cognitive functions at entry into rehabilitation are the least impaired.

Other rate limiters: social cognition

One of the least studied aspects of schizophrenia is emotional functioning, despite the fact that deficits in emotional experience, expression, and perception have been described for almost 100 years. Recently, however, the role of affect and affective information processing in functional outcome has received greater attention. As clearly articulated by Green and colleagues (Green et al, 2000b), a deficit in the ability to process information related to affective factors has the potential to be a major factor in functional outcome. More than in just social domains, affective processing deficits may have wide-ranging impacts on functional outcome.

Social cognition refers to the ability to perceive, interpret, and respond appropriately to affective and other interpersonal cues. In addition, social problem solving, a critical aspect of the maintenance of social and occupational relationships, is also substantially impaired in patients with schizophrenia. It is likely that lower-level aspects of social cognition, such as affect perception and expression, may impact on social interactions as well. For instance, affect perception may be crucial to successful interactions, because the ability to perceive the listener's reaction may be critical for the successful modulation of social and occupational interactions. Socially, being able to determine if the listener is attentive or irritated and then to adjust the topic of conversation may markedly affect the listener's opinion of the speaker. Occupationally, persuasive communication requires the ability to adjust conversations in response to the observable response of the listener, which may have a marked impact on occupational success. Much like cognitive deficits in general, impairments in social cognition appear to be stable over time and very poorly responsive to treatments with antipsychotic medications (Kee et al, 1998).

Furthermore, social cognitive deficits may also make rehabilitation treatment of patients with schizophrenia a slow process (Green and Nuechterlein, 1999).

Summary

Patients with schizophrenia experience deficits in social, occupational, independent living, and self-care skills, with some patients being completely disabled and dependent on others over the course of their entire life. Cognitive deficits appear to be the most consistent predictor of both global and specific aspects of functional outcome in schizophrenia. Even more than any aspect of symptoms, low levels of cognitive performance appear to be the operative factor in the determination of deficits in adaptive life functioning in patients with schizophrenia. While global functional deficit is predicted by many different cognitive deficits, there are some patterns of specific prediction as well. Declarative memory, executive functioning, working memory and vigilance have different patterns of correlation with various aspects of functional outcome. In contrast, intellectual functioning is not particularly associated with functional outcome. As noted in Chapter 3, intellectual functioning is consistently less impaired in patients with schizophrenia than other aspects of cognitive functioning. Patients with essentially average IQ scores can have memory deficits at the level seen in amnestic conditions. In addition, cognitive deficits are also known to slow the rate of learning and reduce the amount of benefit that patients experience from rehabilitation. Deficits in social cognition may also interfere with social and occupational functioning, by limiting patients' ability to perceive social and interpersonal cues.

The implications of these findings are that cognitive deficits are probably the most important target for intervention in patients with schizophrenia. Moreover, these implications are wide-ranging and include the cost of the illnesses and changes associated with aging. These issues are addressed in detail in the rest of the book, ending with discussions of newly developing treatment options for reducing cognitive deficits.

References

Bailer J, Brauner W, Rey ER. Premorbid adjustment as predictor of outcome in schizophrenia: results of a prospective study. *Acta Psychiatrica Scand* 1996; **93**: 368–77.

Bellack AS, Mueser KT, Gingerich S, Agresta J. *Social skills training for schizophrenia: a step-by-step guide.* Guilford Press, New York, 1997.

Bowen L, Wallace CJ, Glynn SM et al. Schizophrenic individuals' cognitive functioning and performance in interpersonal interactions and social skills training procedures. *J Psychiatric Res* 1994; **28**: 289–301.

Breier A, Schreiber JL, Dyer J, Pickar D. National Institute of Mental Health follow-up study of schizophrenia: prognosis and predictors of outcome. *Arch Gen Psychiatry* 1991; **48**: 239–46.

Green MF. What are the functional consequences of neurocognitive deficits in schizophrenia? *Am J Psychiatry* 1996; **153**: 321–30.

Green MF, Kern RS, Braff D et al. Neurocognition and functional outcome in schizophrenia: are we measuring the right stuff? *Schizophr Bull* 2000a; **26**: 119–36.

Green MF, Kern RS, Robertson MJ et al. Relevance of neurocognitive deficits for functional outcome in schizophrenia. In: Sharma T, Harvey PD, eds. *Cognition in schizophrenia.* Oxford: Oxford University Press, 2000b, 178–92.

Green MF, Nuechterlein KH. Should schizophrenia be treated as a neurocognitive disorder? *Schizophr Bull* 1999; **25**: 309–19.

Harvey PD, Howanitz E, Parrella M et al. Symptoms, cognitive functioning, and adaptive skills in geriatric patients with lifelong schizophrenia: a comparison across treatment sites. *Am J Psychiatry* 1998; **155**: 1080–6.

Heaton RK, Pendleton MG. Use of neuropsychological tests to predict patients' everyday functioning. *J Con Consult Psychol* 1981; **49**: 807–21.

Hegarty JD, Baldessanni RJ, Tohen M. One hundred years of schizophrenia: a meta-analysis of the outcome literature. *Am J Psychiatry* 1994; **151**: 1409–16.

Ho B-C, Andreasen N, Flaum M. Dependence on public financial support early in the course of schizophrenia. *Psychiatr Serv* 1997; **48**: 948–50.

Johnstone EC, Owens DG, Bydder GM et al. The spectrum of structural changes in schizophrenia: age of onset as a predictor of cognitive and clinical impairments and their cerebral correlates. *Psychol Med* 1989; **19**: 91–103.

Kee KS, Kern RS, Marshall BD Jr, Green MF. Risperidone versus haloperidol for perception of emotion in treatment-resistant schizophrenia: preliminary findings. *Schizophr Res* 1998; **31**: 159–65.

Keefe RSE, Mohs RC, Losonczy M et al. Socio-sexual functioning and long-term outcome in schizophrenia. *Am J Psychiatry* 1989; **146**: 206–11.

Keefe RSE, Mohs RC, Losonczy MF et al. Characteristics of very poor outcome schizophrenia. *Am J Psychiatry* 1987; **144**: 889–95.

Kern RS, Green MF, Satz P. Neuropsychological predictors of skills training for schizophrenic patients. *Psychiatry Res* 1992; **43**: 223–30.

Langfelt G. *The prognosis in schizophrenia and factors influencing the course of the disease.* Copenhagen: Munksgaard, 1937.

Lieberman JA. Is schizophrenia a neurodegenerative disorder? A clinical and neurobiological perspective. *Biol Psychiatry* 1999; **46**: 729–39.

Meltzer HY, Rabinowitz J, Lee MA et al. Age at onset and gender of schizophrenics in relation to neuroleptic resistance. *Am J Psychiatry* 1997; **154**: 475–82.

Mueser KT. Cognitive functioning, social adjustment, and long-term outcome in schizophrenia. In: Sharma T, Harvey PD, eds. *Cognition in schizophrenia.* Oxford: Oxford University Press, 2000, 157–77.

Mueser KT, Bellack AS, Douglas MS, Wade JH. Prediction of social skill acquisition in schizophrenic and major affective disorder patients from memory and symptomatology. *Psychiatry Res* 1991; **37**: 281–96.

Mueser KT, Drake RE, Bond GR. Recent advances in psychiatric rehabilitation for patients with severe mental illness. *Harvard Rev Psychiatry* 1997; **5**: 123–37.

Perlick D, Mattis S, Stanstny, Teresi J. Neuropsychological discriminators of long-term inpatient or outpatient status in chronic schizophrenia. *J Neuropsychiatry Clin Neurosci* 1992; **4**: 428–34.

Robinson DG, Werner MG, Alvir JM et al. Predictors of treatment response from a first episode of schizophrenia or schizoaffective disorder. *Am J Psychiatry* 1999; **156**: 544–9.

Stern RG, Mohs RC, Davidson M et al. A longitudinal study of Alzheimer's Disease: measurement, rate and predictors of cognitive deterioration. *Am J Psychiatry* 1994; **151**: 390–6.

Swanson CL Jr, Gur RC, Bilker W et al. Premorbid educational attainment in schizophrenia: association with symptoms, functioning, and neurobehavioral measures. *Biol Psychiatry* 1998; **44**: 739–47.

Velligan DI, Mahurin RK, Diamond PL et al. The functional significance of symptomatology and cognitive function in schizophrenia. *Schizophr Res* 1997; **25**: 21–31.

Wieselgren IM, Lindstrom LH. A prospective 1–5 year outcome study in first admitted and readmitted schizophrenic patients. Relationship to heredity, premorbid adjustment, duration of disease and education level at index admission and neuroleptic treatment. *Acta Psychiatrica Scand* 1996; **93**: 9–19

The cost of cognitive impairment in schizophrenia

8

Schizophrenia is the most expensive psychiatric illness and one of the most expensive illnesses overall in terms of total health care costs. Patients with schizophrenia use a disproportionately high amount of health care services. The prevalence of schizophrenia in America is approximately 1% of the entire population, but annual US mental health care expenditures for the treatment of schizophrenia have been estimated to be higher than 2.5% of the total cost of health care, including preventative interventions, in the entire country (Rupp and Keith, 1993). Although schizophrenia affects fewer persons than other mental illnesses, including depression and anxiety, the rate of institutionalization and repeated hospitalization is relatively high and the productivity losses for schizophrenic patients living in the community are also greatly elevated. For example, US estimates for total costs for the treatment of schizophrenia for the year 1994 were approximately $45 billion, or 25% of the total estimated costs of treatment of all mental illnesses. Direct costs for schizophrenia were $24 billion, or slightly more than 50% of total costs for the illness. Annual morbidity and mortality costs were estimated to be $15 billion and $2 billion, respectively. Therefore, it appears that schizophrenia produces a large morbidity and a small but significant mortality. 'Other related costs' for schizophrenia (crime, social welfare administration, incarceration, and family care giving) were $4.5 billion, or close to 60% of 'other related costs' for all mental illnesses (Rice, 1999). Family care giving comprised the most costly item included in this category for schizophrenia.

There are two components of the societal cost of an illness, the direct cost and the indirect cost (Gunderson and Mosher, 1975). Estimation of the direct costs for the treatment of a mental illness is the product of the number and type of mental health services utilized and the estimated price for each type of service. Direct costs are usually those associated with expenditures for diagnosis and treatment such as hospital costs, drugs, outpatient office visits, rehabilitation, and other professional services. Indirect costs are usually confined to the earnings that are not obtained on account of illness, on the part of either the patient or others who are required to assist the patient. This type of formulation often referred to as 'human capital approach' to valuing life, in which healthy human beings are evaluated in terms of their productivity as labour resources.

Indirect costs of an illness include both morbidity and mortality. Morbidity is defined as the value of reduced or lost productivity based on the impairments related to the lifetime effect of mental disorders on an individual's current income, taking into account the timing of onset of the illness, and the duration of the disorder. Mortality is the value of potential lifetime earnings lost by those who died prematurely because of a mental disorder.

Since average life expectancy of individuals in the US and Western Europe extends past the typical retirement age, any death before retirement age leads to an increase in mortality-related costs. Other costs included in estimations of the cost of a mental illness include public and private expenditures for the consequences of crime, productivity losses for individuals incarcerated in prison as a result of a conviction for a mental-illness related crime, and the value of time spent by others to care for family members with a mental illness. Although the American legal system routinely seeks costs for 'pain and suffering' associated with accidents, a financial estimate for reduction in quality of life and psychic pain is usually not entered into typical cost equations. Thus, all of the calculated costs of schizophrenia are directly reflected in terms of expenditures made and earnings lost. As a result, there is no inflation in these estimates based on failure to make occupational progress (upward social mobility) and they completely ignore the reductions in quality of life that would be associated with reduction in disability for patients with schizophrenia.

Another difficult issue for which to

establish a cost basis is that of medical co-morbidity. Many patients with schizophrenia fail to seek health care spontaneously and most do not have regular contact with a primary care physician. As a result, relatively minor medical conditions can worsen from lack of routine attention, leading to the need for more expensive interventions. Due to lack of contact with primary care physicians, little preventive care is offered to patients with schizophrenia, leading many patients to use emergency room services for most health care, including routine matters. It is difficult to estimate the impact of medical co-morbidity on overall health care costs, but these costs are likely to be substantial. Emergency room costs are at least 10 times as high per service unit as an office visit to a primary care physician or nurse practitioner.

Components of the direct cost of schizophrenia

Inpatient services

Acute psychiatric services are highly utilized by patients with schizophrenia. Patients with schizophrenia occupy approximately 25% of all hospital beds (Terkelsen and Menikoff 1995), and constitute the group with the most frequent inpatient admissions (Geller 1992). Patients with schizophrenia represent one-half of all inpatient admissions. For example, in a study examining claims for all reimbursable

medical services in the State of Georgia (Martin and Miller, 1998), it was demonstrated that 10% of a group of patients with schizophrenia had a least one hospitalization within 2 years and a readmission rate of 24% over these 2 years. Although inpatient episodes accounted for a relatively small number of occurrences for these patients, these inpatient stays are extremely expensive and consumed 18% of the total mental health services used by this subset of patients.

Hospitalization costs as estimated by this study are actually a gross underestimate of the total cost of inpatient and institutional treatment of schizophrenia. Long-stay hospital costs were not included because this agency did not pay for long-stay psychiatric hospitalizations. Thus, the patients with the longest (and most expensive) stays are not even included in this database and only patients with a better lifetime course of illness receiving relatively infrequent and abbreviated inpatient stays are included. Long-stay treatments cost as much as $750.00 per day and patients who stay longer than 6 weeks as an inpatient in the current systems of care are likely to stay hospitalized for as long as 20 years.

Outpatient services

There is also evidence that even community-dwelling patients with schizophrenia are heavy utilizers of mental health services (Bartels et al, 1997). The majority of mental health services in the study described above involved some form of regular, every-day treatment, such as day and partial hospitalization. Sixty percent of all of the patients participating in these every-day services had schizophrenia. It is not at all clear from this study which patient variables are associated with type of services received. For instance, it would seem that patients who receive every-day outpatient treatment would be likely to have poor premorbid functioning, severe cognitive deficits, and a lengthy history of social and occupational failures. Thus, it is reasonable to expect that cognitive impairment is a major contributor to higher use of every-day services. After all, cognitive impairment predicts unemployment and patients who work full time would not be attending a full-time day program.

Despite the high costs associated with mental health services in schizophrenia, it is actually a minority of patients with the illness who receive any services at all. Approximately 50% of a large sample of individuals with a psychiatric diagnosis received few mental health services of any kind, including medical monitoring visits (Roth et al, 1997), while approximately 10% of the sample received voluminous amounts of highly individualized services. Patients in the high user group were more likely to have schizophrenia than any other diagnosis. In general, schizophrenia is

under-represented in the group of patients receiving low levels of services (an average of 10 h a year) and over-represented in clusters receiving greater amounts of service. Yet, despite these extremely high cost estimates, most individuals in the US with a diagnosis of schizophrenia have not had contact with a mental health professional in the past year. The differences across illnesses in the level of service used appear stable over the lifespan of people with schizophrenia, in that higher levels of outpatient service use are found on the part of elderly individuals with schizophrenia than those with affective disorders. These elderly patients with schizophrenia are also more disabled in general and more likely to require acute inpatient treatment as well.

A major component of outpatient care for patients with schizophrenia is medication. Older medications have a relatively modest cost, as little as $0.05 per day. Newer medications, including clozapine, risperidone, olanzapine, ziprasidone, and quetiapine, have much higher costs, which can range as high as $18.00 or more per day. Several studies have demonstrated that newer medications are at least as cost effective as older medications and that these medications are actually equally or even less expensive from the perspective of total costs (Essock et al, 2000). These conclusions are based on the finding that use of newer medications is associated with marked reductions in the need for inpatient stays and better functioning in the community between stays (Albright et al, 1996; Chouinard and Albright, 1997; Meltzer et al, 1993). As noted below, other aspects of the effects of these medications may have the potential to reduce the indirect costs of the illness.

Nursing home care

Another major issue is that of the use of nursing home care for patients with schizophrenia. As many patients with schizophrenia are elderly and the illness does not usually improve in late life, large numbers of formerly institutionalized patients with schizophrenia now reside in nursing homes and have high levels of disability (Harvey et al, 1998). In fact, as many as 300 000 patients with schizophrenia may reside in these homes (Goldman et al, 1986), with most of these homes not delivering mental health services on a regular basis (Burns et al, 1993). Thus, there may be more patients with schizophrenia living in institutional care now than at any time in the history of mental health treatment of schizophrenia, while most of these patients do not receive even rudimentary mental health treatment.

Thus, nursing home care may be a major 'hidden cost' for schizophrenia, in that the diagnosis of record of many of these individuals is not schizophrenia. This cost may be enormous, because the total number of patients receiving nursing home care in year 2000 (~300 000) may be as large as the number of institutionalized patients in chronic psychiatric hospitals in 1948 (~275 000). For example, in the US, the typical cost of care in a modest nursing home is around $75.00 per day. This translates into a daily cost of over $20 million for the 300 000 patients who reside in these homes and an annual cost of $7.5 billion. Since many chronic patients are referred to nursing home care at very young ages (often as young as age 55 years), the length of time for which they will receive nursing home care may be substantial.

Indirect costs of schizophrenia
Prevalence of unemployment

The most substantial aspect of the indirect cost of schizophrenia is impairments in employment. Schizophrenia markedly impairs the ability to work. Estimates of permanent and intractable unemployment in schizophrenic patients in developed countries range from 60% to 75%, with the majority of patients who work at all employed part-time in supported employment (Mulkern and Maderscheid, 1989). In fact, only 10% of patients with schizophrenia work full-time in unsupported employment and only about 15% of patients are able to work part-time in unsupported employment.

Additionally, the onset of schizophrenia is associated with a significant decline in functioning compared to premorbid levels of intellectual, social, and occupational performance. The degree of decline exceeds that of psychotic mood disorder. For example, 75% of patients with schizophrenia who have been ill for at least 25 years evidence a downward occupational drift compared to premorbid occupational status. The comparable figures are about 40% for schizoaffective subjects and 30% for affective disordered subjects. Conversely, the proportion of patients with schizophrenia who experience an upward mobility in occupational levels from premorbid levels is less than 10%, compared to 20% of mood disordered patients (Marneros et al, 1992). Premature retirement is also more prevalent in schizophrenic patients. These comparative figures are based on mood disorder comparison groups with histories of psychotic illness, arguing against psychotic symptoms as a rate-limiting factor in occupational outcome in schizophrenia.

Costs of unemployment in schizophrenia

In addition to the human cost of under-employment or unemployment such as diminished quality of life and self-satisfaction, the economic burden on society resulting from impaired work function in schizophrenic patients is significant. The largest contributor to the indirect cost of schizophrenia is failure to work, which is estimated to be at least $15 billion annually (Rice, 1999). This amount reflects the loss of income because of unemployment, loss of tax revenue, and the cost of federal financial support such as social security income. Furthermore, since schizophrenia interferes with education, this lost income is being costed as if the patients had greatly limited earning potential (i.e. close to minimum wage). During periods of economic prosperity, minimum wage labour is largely absent, with most employed individuals receiving pay at considerably more than the minimum wage. In addition, most individuals work in minimum wage jobs for limited periods of time, before they experience upward mobility to better, higher paying jobs. Thus, the true level of indirect cost of schizophrenia is probably 2 to 3 times that earlier estimate.

Disability has a rapid onset in schizophrenia. In fact, at an average of 7 months after first hospitalization over half of schizophrenic patients are primarily supported by social service agencies. Once such support is initiated, it is rarely ever terminated (Ho et al, 1997). Therefore, dependence on public financial support begins early in the course of illness for most hospitalized patients with schizophrenia. For example, over 50% of Veterans Affairs' (VA) patients with a diagnosis of schizophrenia are receiving disability payments from either Social Security or the Department of Veterans Affairs (Rosenheck et al, 1999) and few will ever leave that disability status.

An additional cost of unemployment in schizophrenia is the failure to have health insurance. Most patients with schizophrenia receive largely ambulatory services, focused on medications. The costs of these medications is greater than in the past, but is still not inconsistent with preventative medication treatment received by many employed individuals. Examples of preventative medication treatment include antihypertensives and lipid reducing compounds. The daily cost of atorvastatin and lisinopril may reach that of the most expensive antipsychotic, but the majority of people taking these medications pay for them from their employment-related health insurance. Consequently, an additional component of the indirect cost of schizophrenia is the inability to cover the cost of treatments for conditions that are completely unrelated to the primary psychotic condition. These costs are not considered in many cost models of schizophrenia.

Unemployment in schizophrenia, however, has even more costs. For example, the cost of family care giving to patients with schizophrenia is estimated to be $3.5 billion annually. Patient employment would presumably free some of the time and effort required of family members for their care and would lower this cost estimate. Additionally, employment has been demonstrated to diminish utilization of outpatient and inpatient psychiatric services, thereby reducing direct costs for the illness. For example, in outpatients who utilized services at a mental health centre, the cost of psychiatric treatment services for unemployed patients was over $2,000 per month. Patients at the same clinics who were working part-time, however, used less than half the amount of treatment services, at a mean monthly cost of $910 (Polak and Warner, 1996).

These estimates are consistent with data reported above indicating that high utilizers of outpatient services are often unemployed, and seeking rehabilitation and other services to improve functional outcome. Also, the cost savings in service use associated with employment in schizophrenia is likely to be associated with a number of factors. For example, several studies have randomly assigned unemployed patients to one of two conditions, one in which they received money for work, and the other a volunteer position. At the end of the 6 months, paid subjects demonstrated significantly improved positive symptoms and reduced rehospitalization rates. Thus, the direct benefits of work will likely contribute to reduced direct service use costs.

Contributors to occupational disability

Cognitive impairment and unemployment in schizophrenia

The presence and severity of positive symptoms have generally been believed to be significant determinants of outcome in schizophrenia. However, as noted in the previous chapter, persistent psychotic symptoms contribute negligibly to functional status, including poor work outcomes (Strauss and Carpenter, 1974; Massel et al, 1990; Perlick et al, 1992). In fact, the weight of the evidence suggests that severity of specific clinical symptoms is not related to unemployment and is not a major obstacle to work. Rather, there is increasing evidence that cognitive impairments, and not positive symptoms, are a major determinant of outcome in schizophrenia, including unemployment.

A recent comprehensive review of the literature examining the relationships between clinical symptoms, neurocognitive functioning, and the outcome domains of community functioning (independent living skills, vocational status, quality of life), social skills, and skill acquisition concluded that neurocognitive abilities were more strongly linked to these areas of outcome whereas clinical symptoms were not (Green, 1996). As reviewed in Chapter 7, specific cognitive areas have emerged as more important in the prediction of functional outcome, and they are executive functioning, vigilance, and verbal learning and memory. Verbal memory demonstrated the most consistent relationship between neurocognitive and functional outcome for all three functional outcome domains. Executive functioning demonstrated the strongest relationship with community functioning, which included occupational functioning, quality of life, and independent living skills. It is intuitively clear that the ability to solve problems and to encode and recall verbal information would be useful for the ability to live in the community, to work, as well as to succeed in psychiatric rehabilitation and interpersonal relationships. Unfortunately, schizophrenic patients generally demonstrate serious deficits in executive functioning and verbal memory, which are the likely explanation for life-long occupational disability in patients with schizophrenia even with successful treatment of psychotic symptoms.

The evidence for the relationship between cognitive dysfunction and unemployment is accumulating. A relationship between executive functioning, as measured by the Wisconsin Card Sorting Test (WCST), and work skills demonstrated in a vocational rehabilitation program, has been found repeatedly. Verbal learning and memory and global outcome scores, as measured by the Strauss-Carpenter scale, have been found to be strongly associated (McGurk and Meltzer,

2000). A recent large-scale study examined the relationship between cognition, symptoms, and work status in a group of 243 schizophrenic patients, 39 of whom were employed or volunteering for at least 20 h per week and 206 who were unemployed for at least a year (Meltzer and McGurk, 1999). The groups did not differ in age, gender, or age of illness onset. Additionally, those patients who were employed had significantly better performance on the WCST and on a verbal list learning test. After adjusting for duration of illness and Brief Psychiatric Rating Scale (BPRS) Positive symptom scores, performance on the cognitive assessments remained higher for those patients who were employed. When patients with schizophrenia who were stably employed or in school full-time were compared to patients who were unemployed or employed only part-time, the employed patients performed significantly better than the unemployed patients on measures of executive functioning, working memory and vigilance, and significantly better than the part-time employed group on measures of vigilance and executive functioning. Clinical symptoms, however, were not found to be significantly related to work status. Thus, executive functioning and verbal learning and memory once again proved to be strong correlates of work status, independent of positive symptoms. Overall, these studies indicate that cognitive functioning, in particular, executive functioning, verbal memory, and attention, is a significant correlate of employment in schizophrenia patients, and, that clinical symptoms are not. Thus, the costs aimed at the treatment of psychotic symptoms in schizophrenia are not likely to affect the indirect cost of the illness, because severity of psychotic symptoms does not influence the factors that impair work functioning: cognitive deficits.

Conclusions

Direct costs of schizophrenia are largely inflated by inpatient treatment and are reduced by the use of newer medications with higher compliance, greater relapse prevention, and greater efficacy against positive, negative, and cognitive symptoms of schizophrenia (see Chapter 12). Indirect costs of schizophrenia are largely associated with low rates of employment. Employment in schizophrenia is interfered with largely by deficits in cognitive functioning, not by psychotic symptoms. Cognitive enhancement, as described in Chapters 12 and 13, is a promising strategy to improve the odds of a patient with schizophrenia sustaining higher levels of employment, with both novel antipsychotic medications and additional 'add-on' therapies showing the ability to enhance cognition.

The new antipsychotic medications are likely to have a major impact on reducing the cost of schizophrenia, because of their greater ability to affect both direct costs (through reduction of inpatient stay) and indirect costs (by improving cognitive functioning). Yet, there is a naïve tendency to avoid or require excessive justification for the use of newer medications because of their unit cost and because of a failure of many clinicians and policy-makers to consider the indirect side of the cost equation. The reluctance to use new medications because of their cost ignores the fact that their use has the potential to reduce costs on both sides of the equation. Focusing on reduction of positive symptoms and ignoring employment and other dimensions of functional status addresses only half of the symptom profile in schizophrenia. Psychiatric nomenclature reinforces this perspective, by designating patients whose hallucinations are reduced as 'treatment-responsive', even if the patients are still receiving disability payments and not engaging in work or social activities. The best intervention to reduce total cost in schizophrenia will be able to reduce both psychotic symptoms and cognitive impairments, with the specific cost of this intervention very likely to be justified by its impact. Newer antipsychotic medications are showing promise of being this type of intervention and their effects will likely be augmented by future developments in cognitive enhancement.

References

Albright PS, Livingstone S, Keegan DL et al. Reduction of healthcare resource utilization and costs following the use of risperidone for patients with schizophrenia previously treated with standard antipsychotic therapy: a retrospective analysis using the Saskatchewan Health linkable databases. *Clin Drug Invest* 1996; **11**: 289–99.

Bartels SJ, Mueser KT, Miles KM. Functional impairments in elderly patients with schizophrenia and major affective disorders living in the community: social skills, living skills, and behavior problems. *Behavior Ther* 1997; **28**: 43–63.

Burns BJ, Wagner HR, Taube JE, Magaziner J. Mental health service use by the elderly in nursing homes. *Am J Pub Health* 1993; **83**: 331–7.

Chouinard G, Albright PS. Economic and health state utility determinations for schizophrenic patients treated with risperidone or haloperidol. *J Clin Psychopharmacol* 1997; **17**: 298–307.

Essock SM, Frisman LK, Covell NH, Hargreaves WA. Cost-effectiveness of clozapine compared with conventional antipsychotic medication for patients in state hospitals. *Arch Gen Psychiatry* 2000; **57**: 987–94.

Geller JL. An historical perspective on the role of state hospitals viewed from the 'revolving door'. *Am J Psychiatry* 1992, **149**: 1526–33.

Goldman HH, Feder J, Scanlon W. Chronic mental patients in nursing homes: Reexamining data from the National Nursing Home Survey. *Hosp Community Psychiatry* 1986; **37**: 269–72.

Green MF. What are the functional consequences of neurocognitive deficits in schizophrenia? *Am J Psychiatry* 1996; **153**: 321–30.

Gunderson JG, Mosher LR. The cost of schizophrenia. *Am J Psychiatry* 1975; **132:** 901–6.

Harvey PD, Howanitz E, Parrella M et al. Cognitive, adaptive, and symptomatic features of schizophrenia in late life: a comparison across treatment sites. *Am J Psychiatry* 1998; **155:** 1080–6.

Ho B-C, Andreasen N, Flaum M. Dependence on public financial support early in the course of schizophrenia. *Psychiatr Serv* 1997; **48:** 948–50.

Marneros A, Deister A, Rohde A. Comparison of long-term outcome of schizophrenic, affective, and schizoaffective disorders. *Br J Psychiatry* 1992; **161(S18):** 44–51.

Martin BC, Miller LS. Expenditures for treating schizophrenia: a population-based study of Georgia Medicaid recipients. *Schizphr Bull* 1998; **24:** 439–88.

Massel HK, Liberman RP, Mintz J et al. Re-evaluating the capacity to work of the mentally ill. *Psychiatry* 1990; **53:** 31–43.

McGurk SR, Meltzer HY. The role of cognitive functioning in vocational outcome in schizophrenia. *Schizophr Res* 2000; **45:** 175–84.

Meltzer HY, McGurk SR. The effects of clozapine, risperidone and olanzapine on cognitive functioning in schizophrenia. *Schizophr Bull* 1999; **25:** 233–55.

Meltzer HY, Cola P, Way L et al. Cost effectiveness of clozapine in neuroleptic-resistant schizophrenia. *Am J Psychiatry* 1993; **150:** 1630–8.

Mulkern VM, Maderscheid RW. Characteristics of community support program clients in 1980 and 1984. *Hosp Community Psychiatry* 1989; **40:** 165–72.

Perlick D, Mattis S, Stastny P, Teresi J. Neuropsychological discriminators of long-term inpatient or outpatient status in chronic schizophrenia. *J Neuropsychiatry Clin Neurosci* 1992; **4:** 428–34.

Polak P, Warner R. The economic life of seriously mentally ill people in the community. *Psychiatr Serv* 1996; **47:** 270–3.

Rice DP. Economic burden of mental disorders in the United States. *Econ Neurosci* 1999; **1:** 40–4.

Rosenheck R, Frisman L, Kasprow W. Improving access to disability benefits among homeless persons with mental illness: an agency-specific approach to services integration. *Am J Public Health* 1999; **89:** 524–8.

Roth D, Lauber BG, Crane-Ross D, Clark JA. Impact of mental health reform on patterns of service delivery. *Community Ment Health J* 1997; **33:** 473–86.

Rupp A, Keith SJ. The costs of schizophrenia. Assessing the burden. *Psychiatr Clin North Am* 1993; **16:** 913–23.

Strauss JS, Carpenter WT Jr. Characteristic symptoms and outcome in schizophrenia. *Arch Gen Psychiatry* 1974; **30:** 429–34.

Terkelsen KG, Menikoff A. Measuring the costs of schizophrenia. Implications for the post-institutional era in the US. *Pharmacoeconomics* 1995; **8:** 199–222.

Cognitive and functional changes with aging

9

The cognitive correlates of aging in schizophrenia have been a neglected topic, much like the study of other aspects of schizophrenia in late life. Cognitive and functional changes occur with normal aging in the population as a whole, particularly after the age of 70 years. This raises the question as to the status of cognitive and functional performance in individuals with a life-long history of cognitive compromise, such as patients with schizophrenia. Since patients with schizophrenia have profound deficits early in life, what would be the level of functioning seen after a lifetime of illness? A further question is that of the interaction between degenerative conditions that occur most frequently in late life and schizophrenia. It is important not to mistake changes in cognitive or functional status caused by illnesses such as Alzheimer's disease for changes associated with the course of schizophrenia in late life.

There is evidence that variability in the outcome and cognitive status of elderly patients with schizophrenia may, if anything, be greater than in younger patients. Since functional status is determined, in large part, by cognitive functioning (see Chapters 7 and 8), one would expect substantial variations in cognitive functioning across patients with a history of different lifetime courses of illness. Although some elderly individuals with a history of schizophrenia are apparently symptom-free and have little residual deficit in late life (Harding et al, 1987), many patients with a lifelong history of chronic schizophrenia either have lengthy stays in chronic care (Davidson et al, 1995) or have extensive adaptive deficit (Bartels et al, 1997) while living in the community either after de-institutionalization from extended hospital stays or between episodes. Several studies of the cognitive and functional characteristics of patients with late-onset schizophrenia following a lifetime of adequate adaptive skills have suggested no evidence of increasing impairment with age (Jeste et al, 1995). However, these patients have not had an entire lifetime of experiencing the symptoms and treatments associated with schizophrenia.

Patients whose lifetime outcome was generally good, not consisting of either institutional stays or continuous illness while living in the community, appear to have minimal evidence of cognitive change in later life (Eyler Zorrilla et al, 2000; Heaton et al, 1994; 2001). These older good-outcome patients with schizophrenia have been reported not to show increased cognitive impairment compared to age-corrective normative standards, relative to younger patients with schizophrenia. It is not that these patients have no impairments in their cognitive functioning. Most of these patients

had significant levels of impairment and as many as 70% would be seen to meet clinical criteria for 'substantial neuropsychological deficit' (Palmer et al, 1997). Thus, considerable cognitive and functional deficit persists in patients with lifelong schizophrenia, even in patients whose relative level of lifelong functional disability is relatively mild and whose relative impairment has not worsened compared to younger patients. These patients with a lifetime of good outcome may not show marked evidence of decline above and beyond changes expected from normal aging processes (Heaton et al, 2001). However, there are some limitations in the studies from which these impressions come. The primary limitation of these studies is that the majority of the patients in these studies are actually not particularly old and they are clearly younger than the poor outcome patients who have been the subject of most longitudinal studies on cognitive change in older patients with schizophrenia.

There are, however, a substantial number of patients whose global functional status is markedly impaired over the course of their entire lifetime. In the past, these patients might have been institutionalized for life. As noted in the last chapter, many states have begun the process of closing their state hospitals or converting them into exclusively forensic facilities and it is estimated that at least 300 000 patients with lifelong chronic schizophrenia have been referred to nursing homes as a part of this de-institutionalization movement (Bartels et al, 1997; Strahan, 1990). As a result, even though the overall number of patients who experience extended psychiatric hospital stays into late life is reduced, there are many schizophrenic patients receiving institutional care of some type in their later life. Since these patients are quite likely to have had severe cognitive and functional deficits earlier in their lives, their current status may be marked by even greater impairments in these areas.

There is also evidence that these same poor outcome patients may have a differential likelihood of experiencing deterioration in brain structure over time compared to better outcome patients. As described in the next chapter, progressive ventricular enlargement is found in patients with chronic, treatment-refractory positive symptoms of schizophrenia. This deterioration in brain structure may have direct implications for progressive changes in cognitive and functional status in later life as well. Middle-aged poor outcome patients have been found to have progressive increases in ventricular size over 3-year (Mathalon et al, 2001) and 5-year follow-up studies (Davis et al, 1998). If this progression of ventricular change were to continue over the course of their later years as well, the cumulative effects of these changes could be substantial.

Comparisons of cognitive functioning in good and poor outcome patients

Direct comparative studies are rare at this time, but some data from standardized assessments that would allow for comparisons have been collected that would allow for some inferences. Geriatric patients in the age range of 65–85 years with schizophrenia who were either acutely admitted patients with a good lifetime functional outcome or chronically institutionalized patients differed substantially in cognitive and functional status (Harvey et al, 1998). Acutely admitted patients, although not differing from chronic patients in the severity of their psychotic symptoms, outperformed the institutionalized patients by 12 points on the Mini Mental State Examination (MMSE) and by over a full standard deviation on a neuropsychological assessment composite score. Since the good outcome patients themselves underperformed normative standards by about 1.5 SD, this suggests significant cognitive impairment on the part of the poor outcome patients. Adaptive deficits were also more severe in the poor outcome patients, although the correlates of these functional deficits were the same in good and bad outcome patients. In both groups, cognitive performance deficit was the best predictor of adaptive functioning deficit.

When levels of cognitive impairment are compared across poor outcome patients

Table 9.1
Descriptive characteristics of good and poor outcome patients with schizophrenia in later life

Lifetime outcome status	*Good*	*Poor*
Level of adaptive deficit	*Moderate*	*Severe*
Course of cognitive and functional status	*Stable*	*Decline in some patients*
Severity of cognitive impairment	*Moderate*	*Severe*
Predictors of adaptive deficit	*Cognitive impairment*	*Cognitive impairment*

studied in different sites, there is remarkable similarity. For instance, poor outcome patients studied in suburban Philadelphia (Arnold et al, 1995) had essentially identical MMSE scores to poor outcome patients studied in New York, as did institutionalized patients in the US and UK; performance in chronically hospitalized patients across the two countries was found to be within one MMSE point (Harvey et al, 1997). These data suggest that idiosyncratic variations in the environment associated with different systems of care are not strongly associated with cognitive functioning. Table 9.1 shows the characteristics of good and poor outcome patients with schizophrenia.

Age effects on cognition in poor outcome patients

Performance on global measures of cognitive functioning such as the MMSE is more deteriorated in older poor outcome patients compared to younger patients. Differences in cognitive performance as large as 3 MMSE points per decade have been found in institutionalized patients across the age range of 25–95 years (Davidson et al, 1995). The average MMSE score of patients between the ages of 85 and 95 years was 9.6 in one study, which is extremely low considering that patients whose scores were 0 on the instrument were excluded from the analysis. Since these findings have been replicated in other sites, these results indicate that deterioration, quite significant in magnitude, in some dimensions of cognitive functioning is occurring in at least some poor outcome patients. These data must be considered in the context that cross-sectional comparisons always exaggerate age-related changes. Yet, even if these results were slightly over-estimating the differences between the oldest and youngest patients, the level of impairment seen in these older patients is so great that there is no chance that this is a consequence of normal aging processes. After all, some research on cognitive functioning in aging has suggested that community-dwelling individuals over the age of 85 years with less than 4 years of formal education score around 20 on the MMSE, a score that is 10 points higher than patients with schizophrenia of the same age with 8 or more years of education (Crum et al, 1993).

Similarity of cognitive deficits in geriatric schizophrenia to degenerative dementia

It was believed that there was an elevated prevalence of Alzheimer's disease in postmortem brain specimens from patients with schizophrenia (Prohovnik et al, 1993). If true, this finding would suggest that the profound impairments seen in older patients with schizophrenia were due to some increase in their risk for the development of Alzheimer's disease or some other degenerative condition. In response, several studies have been conducted to examine the profile and course of cognitive deficits in Alzheimer's disease and schizophrenia. In terms of the profile, several studies have found that patients with schizophrenia perform more poorly than patients with Alzheimer's disease on most aspects of a comprehensive neuropsychological battery (Davidson et al,

1996; Heaton et al, 1994). Alzheimer's disease patients, in contrast, were more impaired than schizophrenic patients on delayed recall memory. When directly evaluating the performance of these two patient groups, it was discovered that the schizophrenic patients performed more poorly than the patients with Alzheimer's disease on executive functioning, naming, and motor skills, while the two groups performed equivalently on the rate of verbal learning.

There is very little information available about the course of schizophrenia in late life as compared to the clinical course of Alzheimer's disease. A number of studies, using either cognitive screening measures or comprehensive neuropsychological batteries sensitive to the typical deficits in Alzheimer's disease have found that, as a group, there was no decline in performance over 1- to 2-year follow-ups of elderly patients with schizophrenia (Harvey et al, 1995; 1997). In contrast, patients with Alzheimer's disease have clinically significant cognitive declines during the same 1-year time frame, suggesting a substantially different course of illness than patients with schizophrenia.

Several different neuropathological studies have indicated that patients with schizophrenia do not manifest evidence of the classical postmortem neuropathology of progressive degenerative dementias, such as amyloid plaques, neurofibrillary tangles, Lewy bodies, or alterations in indicators of

Table 9.2
Differential features of Alzheimer's disease (AD) and schizophrenia

	AD	Schizophrenia
Clinical		
Progressive annual decline	Yes	No
Delayed memory impairment	Profound	Moderate
New learning	Impaired	Impaired
Executive functioning	Impaired	More impaired
Biological		
Cholinergic deficits	Yes	No
Plaques and tangles	Yes	Equivalent to normal

acetylcholine activity (Arnold and Trojanowski, 1996; Purohit et al, 1998). These results are similar across research sites, ages of patients, and the level of overall functional deficit seen at the time of death. As a result, the neuropathology and neurobiology of cognition in late-life schizophrenia is still an open question. Table 9.2 contrasts the status of cognitive deficits in schizophrenia and degenerative dementia.

Important issues to consider

Cohort effects

Older patients with schizophrenia are known to have completed less education than younger patients, with the possibility arising that age-related differences in cognitive performance are all due to differences in educational attainment. In terms of the issue of cohort

effects, it is important to keep in mind that the average level of education completed by both the population as a whole and demographically similar patients with schizophrenia is greater in younger individuals than in older ones. As a result, cross-sectional comparisons across wide age ranges almost always exaggerate the level of within-individual change over time. Yet, the effect of education is not great enough to account for the large levels of difference in performance across younger and older patients. The Davidson et al study of younger and older patients has found that the youngest patients in the study (25–34 years) completed 3 more years of education on average than the oldest patients (85–94 years). The difference in MMSE scores between these groups was much larger, with the youngest patients performing 19 points better than the older patients out of a possible total score of 30.

Thus, on the surface it could appear that

differences in education account for these differences in cognitive performance. There are two arguments against this interpretation. The first is that, as noted above, healthy individuals over the age of 85 years with less than 4 years of formal education have been found to have average MMSE scores above 20 (Crum et al, 1993). The second is that some of these older patients manifest a profile of academic achievement that is inconsistent with lifelong cognitive impairment of this magnitude. In one study, eight of the 24 patients over the age of 65 years who had completed college had MMSE scores less than 10 (Davidson et al, 1995). Thus, patients who attended a university had MMSE scores in a range suggestive of profound dementia and essentially no learning potential, indicating quite strongly that this could not be their lifelong level of functioning.

Low baseline performance

Healthy individuals experience some decline in their cognitive capacity with increasing age. These decreases tend to be largest in learning, memory, and attentional functioning and least in long-term memory and reading skills, exactly the same profiles of cognitive deficit that are seen in schizophrenia starting at the onset of the illness. For healthy individuals, there is a decline of as much as 50% in declarative memory performance from age 35 to 75 years (Wechsler, 1987) and, as a result, it is very

important to consider the normative standards for performance of older individuals, before thinking that any change in memory performance signifies an abnormal decline. Furthermore, a healthy individual who loses 50% of their average to superior memory capacity will still be recalling a substantial amount of information in later life. For example, an individual with 50th percentile performance will be remembering 20 out of 50 pieces of information at age 75 in contrast to 40 out of 50 at age 35. What if memory performance at age 35 were consistent with learning only eight out of 50 pieces of information? Performance at age 75 years would involve recalling only four out of 50 and performing well within the demented range.

This last example characterizes patients with schizophrenia. As a result, it is important not to confuse performing very poorly in late life, consistent with lifelong poor performance, from worsening in late life and performing relatively more poorly compared to earlier performance. Poor performance in early life predicts poor performance in later life, with deterioration truly occurring in individuals whose relative performance declines over time compared to their own earlier performance.

The age of patients studied

Some studies of 'older' patients with schizophrenia included patients as young as 45 years (e.g. Eyler Zorilla et al, 2000; Heaton et al, 1994; Heaton et al, 2001). In order to detect normal changes in functioning in healthy individuals, short-term studies would not be able to do so in samples this young. Major changes in healthy individuals' cognitive functioning do not occur with any frequency until after age 60 years. There are serious problems involved in extrapolating from short-term (1 year or thereabouts) studies of younger (age less than at least 60 years) patients with schizophrenia, in terms of detection of abnormal declines in cognitive functioning. The risk of cognitive decline in healthy populations at this age is so minimal that any detectable change in a patient population would have to be enormous by comparison. If cognitive decline in schizophrenia was due to an exaggeration of the normal aging process in individuals who experience long-term compromise, then the age of the subjects studied should be in the range where changes with aging are common and detectable in the healthy population. In addition, even in healthy populations, changes are often not detected at 1-year periods, with 10 or more-year follow-ups more likely to identify within-subject changes (Constantine et al, 1999).

For example, if a sample of 100 healthy 35-year-old individuals were followed up for 1 year and examined for changes in the cognitive functioning, it is quite unlikely that any of these individuals would show any decline in any aspect of their functioning. If the researchers following this sample were willing to extrapolate in the ways that schizophrenia researchers often do from similar studies, then they could reach several preposterous conclusions:

There is no such thing as dementia;
Age-related cognitive change is a myth;
And, finally,
The only cause of death is accidents.

These conclusions are clearly wrong. Yet, they are strictly based on the empirical data collected from the hypothetical 1-year follow-up study. The typical study of cognition in schizophrenia that has led to the conclusion that cognitive functioning is completely stable over the entire lifespan has been a study of patients under the age of 45 years followed for 1 year or less. Since cognitive change, if it occurs, in schizophrenia does not have the rapid and continuous progression seen in Alzheimer's disease, it must be either:

(a)   Insidious over the course of many years and so subtle each year that it would not be detectable. After all, a 3-point per decade change in MMSE scores would only be 0.3 points a year, an amount that is not detectable with the MMSE.

(b)   Distributed across patients, with some limited number of patients showing a modest change each year.

(c)   Absent and not occurring at levels above age-related changes for low functioning individuals.

Evidence regarding progressive decline in individual patients with schizophrenia

Whole sample differences over time in cognitive performance tell us little about the prevalence or rate of individual changes. Even in poor outcome patients who have evidence of previous cognitive decline, it appears clear that year-to-year change is not detected for the group as a whole. However, there are several reasons that individual patients could be declining while the mean scores for the group as a whole do not. First, a number of patients could be manifesting trivial improvements in their performance scores due to practice effects that over-ride larger drops in functioning experienced by a small number of decliners. Second, patients with a declining course might be more likely to be lost to follow-up than non-decliners and this would mask group changes based on assessment of patients who could be followed. Finally, if the number of patients who declined was small enough and the amount of decline was limited enough, an increase in variance at the follow-up assessment might be the only measurable signal for the group as a whole.

There have been three previous follow-up studies for 3 or more years of patients who were over the age of 65 years at the start of the follow-up. In one study, over 300 older patients were followed for 3 years (Harvey et

al, 1999a). At the first follow-up (15–18 months) the risk of cognitive decline was 12.6%. At the second follow-up (30–36 months), an additional 15% met criteria for worsening over the follow-up period, for a total rate of cognitive decline of 27.6%. The risk factors that were associated with increases in risk for cognitive and functional decline included: older age, lower levels of formal education, and more severe positive symptoms at baseline. Gender was not associated with risk for cognitive and functional decline, nor was neuroleptic treatment status, negative symptom severity at the baseline assessment, or age at first psychiatric admission.

A second study (Harvey et al, 1999b) examining 57 patients who were first identified in the chronic care psychiatric hospital, de-institutionalized to nursing home care, and then re-evaluated an average of 30 months later found several changes in cognitive and functional status. Both cognitive functioning (estimated by the MMSE) and scores on functional status were found to decline significantly, while positive and negative symptoms were stable over time. These data indicate that cognitive decline may predict deterioration in overall functional status, consistent with the data from Chapter 7 regarding the correlation of cognitive and adaptive skills and with studies of dementia suggesting that functional decline follows the occurrence of cognitive decline.

In the third study, 108 schizophrenic

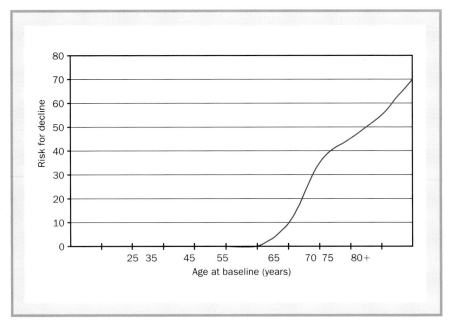

Figure 9.1
Risk for cognitive decline in schizophrenic patients over 6 years as a function of age.

patients ranging in age from 20 to 80 years were followed over 6 years, with the schizophrenic subjects over age 50 years compared to a group of 126 healthy comparison subjects and 118 Alzheimer's disease patients (Friedman et al, 2001). When the risk for cognitive decline was compared across the groups, age-related risks were different in each group. For the Alzheimer's disease patients, over 90% of the patients, regardless of age, manifested a worsening in their cognitive status, in contrast to the healthy subjects who had no risk of worsening regardless of age. Patients with schizophrenia had no risk of worsening until after age 65 years. Patients over the age of 65 years had a consistent age-related increase in risk for decline over the follow-up period. These findings were also replicated with MMSE scores, where Alzheimer's disease patients declined an average of 12 MMSE points over 6 years and the healthy sample had a 1-point change in the oldest patients. In the patients with schizophrenia, no declines were noted until after age 65 years, while the patients over the age of 65 years demonstrated an increase in the extent of worsening from a drop of 2 points over the next 6 years in patients aged 65–69 years, 3 points for ages 70–74 years, and 5 points for ages 75–80 years.

In summary, short-term studies of poor outcome patients with schizophrenia indicate that some of these patients manifest declines in their cognitive and functional status over follow-up periods ranging from 3 to 6 years. These declines are not present in all cases and are associated with age. Figure 3 shows the age-associated risk of cognitive decline in patients with schizophrenia followed up over 6 years. The characteristics of this progression, much like the profiles of impairment previously discussed, are not consistent with the rate of progression seen in degenerative diseases and the lack of concurrent vascular events argues against vascular dementia as a cause of this stepwise change.

There are a number of caveats regarding these findings. First, the patients who have been followed longitudinally and who were over the age of 65 years at entry into the study had a uniformly consistent history of poor lifetime functional outcome. Many of these patients had lived their lives in institutional care. Second, these patients had extensive treatment histories with conventional antipsychotic medications and other invasive treatments such as electroconvulsive therapy

(ECT). While having received these treatments did not correlate with cognitive functioning, the risk for decline may be affected.

Conclusion

Some patients with schizophrenia appear to decline in their cognitive functioning, those being older patients with a lifetime history of poor functional outcome and substantial lifetime cognitive impairment. It is impossible to know if patients over the age of 65 years with a lifetime history of better outcome also decline, because similar longitudinal studies have not been completed. Recent work has indicated that even very poor outcome patients under the age of 65 years do not show evidence of cognitive decline, indicating that this decline is most likely age-related. More severe and treatment-refractory symptoms appear to be a risk factor for this decline. Interestingly, recent research suggests that persistent psychotic symptoms are a risk factor for progressive loss of cortical volume as well. Since poor outcome patients with schizophrenia have been shown to demonstrate progressive ventricular enlargement, the connection between persistent psychotic symptoms and cortical deterioration in middle life may turn out to be related to cognitive decline in later life. Currently, however, the most accurate statement is that a limited subset of patients (i.e. those with lifetime poor functional outcome) are known to decline and information is lacking about the majority of patients. Cognitive decline predicts functional decline, consistent with the relationship between these two variables at the beginning and middle of the course of illness.

References

Arnold SE, Gur RE, Shapiro RM et al. Prospective clinicopathologic studies of schizophrenia: accrual and assessment of patients. *Am J Psychiatry* 1995; **152**: 731–7.

Arnold SE., Trojanowski JQ. Cognitive impairment in elderly schizophrenia: a dementia (still) lacking distinctive histopathology. *Schizophr Bull* 1996; **22**: 5–9.

Bartels SJ, Mueser KT, Miles KM. Functional impairments in elderly patients with schizophrenia and major affective disorders living in the community: social skills, living skills, and behavior problems. *Behavior Ther* 1997; **28**: 43–63.

Constantine G, Lyketsos CG, Chen LS, Anthony JC. Cognitive decline in adulthood: an 11.5-year follow-up of the Baltimore Epidemiologic Catchment Area study. *Am J Psychiatry* 1999; **156**: 58–65.

Crum RM, Anthony JC, Bassett SS, Folstein MF. Population-based norms for the Mini-Mental State Examination by age and educational level. *JAMA* 1993; **269**: 2386–91.

Davidson M, Harvey PD, Powchik P et al. Severity of symptoms in geriatric chronic schizophrenic patients. *Am J Psychiatry* 1995; **152**: 197–207.

Davidson M, Harvey PD, Welsh K et al. Cognitive impairment in old-age schizophrenia: a comparative study of schizophrenia and Alzheimer's disease. *Am J Psychiatry* 1996; **153**: 1274–9.

Davis KL, Buchsbaum MS, Shihabuddin L et al. Ventricular enlargement in poor outcome schizophrenia. *Biol Psychiatry* 1998; **43**: 783–93.

Eyler Zorrilla LT, Heaton RK, McAdams LA et al. Cross-sectional study of older outpatients with schizophrenia and healthy comparison subjects: no differences in age-related cognitive decline. *Am J Psychiatry* 2000; **157**: 1324–6.

Friedman JI, Harvey PD, Coleman T et al. A six-year follow-up across the lifespan in schizophrenia. A comparison with Alzheimer's Disease and health projects. *Am J Psychiatry* 2001; **158**: 1441–8.

Harding CM, Brooks GW, Ashikaga T et al. The Vermont longitudinal study of persons with severe mental illness. II. Long term outcome of subjects who retrospectively met DSM-III criteria for schizophrenia. *Am J Psychiatry* 1987; **144**: 727–35.

Harvey PD, Howanitz E, Parrella M et al. Symptoms, cognitive functioning, and adaptive skills in geriatric patients with lifelong schizophrenia: a comparison across treatment sites. *Am J Psychiatry* 1998; **155**: 1080–6.

Harvey PD, Leff J, Trieman N et al. Cognitive impairment and adaptive deficit in geriatric chronic schizophrenic patients: a cross national study in New York and London. *Int J Geriatr Psychiatry* 1997; **12**: 1001–7.

Harvey PD, Lombardi J, Leibman M et al. Performance of chronic schizophrenic patients on cognitive neuropsychological measures sensitive to dementia. *Int J Geriatr Psychiatry* 1996; **11**: 621–7.

Harvey PD, Moriarty PJ, Friedman JI et al. Differential preservation of cognitive functions in geriatric patients with lifelong chronic schizophrenia: reduced impairment in reading scores compared to other skill areas. *Biol Psychiatry* 2000; **47**: 962–8.

Harvey PD, Parrella M, White L et al. Convergence of cognitive and adaptive decline in late-life schizophrenia. *Schizophr Res* 1999b; **35**: 77–84.

Harvey PD, Silverman JM, Mohs RC et al. Cognitive decline in late-life schizophrenia: a longitudinal study of geriatric chronically hospitalized patients. *Biol Psychiatry* 1999a; **45**: 32–40.

Harvey PD, White L, Parrella M et al. The longitudinal stability of cognitive impairment in schizophrenia. Mini-mental state scores at one and two-year follow-ups in geriatric in-patients. *Br J Psychiatry* 1995;**166**: 630–3.

Heaton RK, Gladsjo JA, Palmer BW et al. Stability and course of neuropsychological deficits in schizophrenia. *Arch Gen Psychiatry* 2001; **58**: 24–32.

Heaton R, Paulsen JS, McAdams LA et al. Neuropsychological deficits in schizophrenics. Relationship to age, chronicity, and dementia. *Arch Gen Psychiatry* 1994; **51**: 469–76.

Jeste DV, Harris MJ, Krull A et al. Late-onset schizophrenia: clinical and neuropsychological characteristics. *Am J Psychiatry* 1995; **172**: 722–30.

Mathalon DH, Sullivan EV, Lim KO, Pfefferbaum A. Progressive brain volume changes and the clinical course of schizophrenia in men: a longitudinal magnetic resonance imaging study. *Arch Gen Psychiatry* 2001; **58**: 148–57.

Palmer BW, Heaton RK, Paulsen JS et al. Is it possible to be schizophrenic yet neuropsychologically normal? *Neuropsychology* 1997; **11**: 437–46.

Purohit DP, Perl DP, Haroutunian V et al. Alzheimer's disease and related neurodegenerative diseases in elderly patients with schizophrenia: a postmortem neuropathology of 100 cases. *Arch Gen Psychiatry* 1998; **55**: 205–11.

Prohovnik I, Dwork AJ, Kaufman MA, Wilson N. Alzheimer-type neuropathology in elderly schizophrenia patients. *Schizophrenia Bulletin* 1993; **19**: 805–16.

Strahan GW. Prevalence of selected mental disorders in nursing and related care homes, in Mental Health, United States, 1990: DHHS Publication ADM 90–1708. Edited by Mandersheid RW, Sonnenschein MA. Washington, DC: US Government Printing Office, 1990.

Wechsler D. *The Wechsler Memory Scales*, revised. San Antonio TX, USA: Psychological Corporation, 1987.

The neuroimaging correlates of cognitive deficits

10

Neuroimaging techniques have revolutionized the study of schizophrenia; findings dating from the 1970s have demonstrated that there are clear brain structural abnormalities associated with the condition (Johnstone, 1976). Recent Magnetic Resonance Imaging (MRI) research has identified brain characteristics associated with the early stages of psychosis and studies, using functional MRI (fMRI), have shown the effects of medication in the brain.

In one set of studies, our research group, the Section on Cognitive Psychopharmacology at the Institute of Psychiatry, London, applied established imaging techniques such as structural MRI to new patient groups, such as people in their earliest stages of psychosis. The findings have shown that structural changes may predate the onset of schizophrenia and may become a useful early indicator for psychosis.

This chapter discusses how findings such as these indicate that neuroimaging techniques may prove useful as biological markers and could ultimately act as aids to diagnosis and treatment selection in schizophrenia.

Biological markers for schizophrenia would greatly aid the diagnostic process and the assessment of treatment response. Indeed, many abnormalities such as ventricular enlargement, dopamine D2 receptor density, amphetamine-stimulated central nervous system dopamine release, plasma homovanillic acid and smooth pursuit eye tracking dysfunction are present in people experiencing their first episode of psychosis who later develop schizophrenia. But in isolation, these 'abnormalities' lack specificity, that is, many are also present in those who do not develop schizophrenia but go on to develop other disorders (Copolov and Crook, 2000). The value of these possible biological markers for schizophrenia may lie in their use in combination.

Understanding how the structure of the brain may be abnormal in schizophrenia has been central to advancing our knowledge of the illness. However, possibly the most exciting advances in schizophrenia research have followed from neuroimaging techniques which facilitate the visualization of brain function. These allow us to investigate the neurochemical and neurovascular systems that may be abnormal in schizophrenia at a global and regional level. This offers the potential to understand how changes in blood flow and metabolic activity may link to the cognitive dysfunction and primary symptoms of schizophrenia, and how these may be affected by antipsychotic medication.

Functional imaging in schizophrenia

There are three modalities that have been used primarily to visualize the brain in action –

Positron Emission Tomography (PET), Single Photon Emission Tomography (SPECT or SPET) and functional Magnetic Resonance Imaging (fMRI).

PET is a technique that facilitates the evaluation of cerebral metabolic activity, blood flow and also allows neurotransmitter receptor quantification and function. However, given the need for an on-site cyclotron unit, it has very limited availability. Cerebral metabolic activity is measured by glucose metabolism using PET. Glucose is the energy currency of neurons, and abnormal glucose metabolism is an indication of underlying pathology. The tracer employed in PET imaging of glucose metabolism is $[^{18}F]$-deoxyglucose. Regional glucose metabolism can be assessed with PET during the resting state, or during performance of a cognitive task by monitoring emissions from the tracer as it is metabolized. The distribution will reflect cerebral glucose utilization under specific pathological or mental conditions. Increased neuronal activity in an area of the brain is paralleled by an increase in blood supply. Regional cerebral blood flow (rCBF) is the technique used to measure this increase in blood blow. Images of rCBF are obtained by using water labelled with an oxygen isotope $[^{15}O]$-H_2O. When a particular region is activated it needs more blood, therefore by tracking the emissions from the radiolabelled water it is possible to track which regions are activated while a person is performing specific cognitive tasks. Single Photon Emission Computed Tomography (SPECT) is a similar technique to PET, and may be used for direct measurement of central neurochemical systems in vivo. It is based on single photon emissions from decaying radionuclides. Like PET, SPECT allows us to study neurotransmitter receptors, the site of action of psychotropic drugs and the functional effects of psychiatric illness and medication on regional brain activity. In terms of comparing the two techniques, SPECT is a cheaper and more widely available technique, as it does not require an on-site cyclotron unit, but it is hampered by lower spatial resolution. Both these techniques use radioactivity and have lower spatial and temporal resolution than functional MRI.

Probably the greatest advance in psychiatric neuroimaging of the last few years has been the development of fMRI. With spatial resolution of as little as 1 mm, and the ability to capture responses in the brain occurring over a period of seconds (although reconstruction and processing of the raw data commonly occurs after scanning), it has proven to be a popular tool in mapping the brain. It is far superior to PET and SPECT and offers the possibility of mapping cognitive function to very precise neuroanatomical structures, helping to identify structures and functional networks which may be abnormal in schizophrenia and other psychiatric illnesses. Thus, since the late 1990s, fMRI has

become the 'procedure of choice' for studying brain function in schizophrenia (Longworth et al, 1999) and has been employed to localize brain regions linked to cognitive deficits and/or symptoms. Recently, it has also proved useful for visualizing treatment response (see Chapter 15).

fMRI detects regions of neuronal activity by monitoring changes in levels of blood oxygenation, and Blood Oxygenation Level Dependent (BOLD) imaging is the most common form of fMRI. Use of this technique relies on the supposition that when neural activity increases, the flow of oxygenated blood to that particular region also increases. Because the supply of oxygenated blood flow outstrips demand for oxygen, it is possible to detect an excess in the amount of oxygenated blood compared with deoxygenated blood. The resulting change in the ratio of deoxyhaemoglobin to oxyhaemoglobin causes an increase in the magnetic resonance signal which is used as a marker of functional activation (Figure 10.1). The signal is then mapped onto the subject's own anatomical scan to indicate the location of increased activity. Data can also be combined across subjects to provide group-averaged images mapped into standard neurological coordinates.

fMRI is a non-invasive and safe technique. It does not require radioactivity, unlike Positron Emission Tomography (PET) or Single Photon Emission Tomography (SPET),

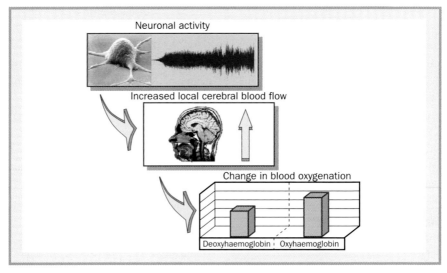

Figure 10.1
*Principles involved in converting neuronal activity into a blood oxygenation level dependent (BOLD) signal,
which can be measured with functional magnetic resonance imaging. Adapted with permission from British
Medical Journal, Longworth et al, 1999.*

and uses the brain's natural haemodynamic
response to neural activity as an endogenous
tracer. It can be carried out during the same
session as a routine MRI scan in a clinical
scanner allowing both structural and functional
information to be collected in the same visit.
The process usually involves measuring the
changes in cerebral blood flow (changes in the
BOLD signal) while people are engaged in
covert or overt responses (Longworth et al,
1999). Thus it is possible to repeat scans on the
same individuals as often as necessary, to allow
the tracking of changes in the brain over time
and to monitor the response to treatment.

Although a promising technique, fMRI's

use is still limited to research for several reasons.
For example, the relationship between the
BOLD signal and brain activation has still not
yet been conclusively elucidated. Assuming that
theoretical assumptions underlying fMRI are
correct, there are still several practical and
technical obstacles to be overcome before the
technique can be clinically useful. Some older
MR machines are not capable of performing
functional imaging. In addition, the use of
fMRI is also still relatively new in
schizophrenia. Sample sizes used are often small
(i.e. under 20 participants) and the variety of
methods used for the analysis of fMRI image
has led to some conflicting results.

Furthermore, the technique can produce artefacts, e.g. movement of subjects in the scanner produces signal changes that mimic changes in neuronal activity (Callicott et al, 1998). Future research to iron out these problems will come from psychological, engineering and biostatistical sciences. In addition to these technical limitations there are other issues of a practical nature, such as the careful screening necessary to ensure that candidates for a scan can tolerate the noise of the scanner and close confinement within the magnet bore, and that they are free of metallic implants.

Visualizing symptoms in schizophrenia

Recent research has examined whether the major symptoms of schizophrenia can be linked to abnormal functioning of one or more brain regions. Answering this question may help to identify how antipsychotics may change brain function leading to a decrease in psychotic symptoms since the older and newer antipsychotics seem to have equivalent effects on psychotic symptoms.

In a landmark paper, Liddle et al (1992) investigated the links between patterns of rCBF and symptoms. They identified three primary symptom clusters, psychomotor poverty, disorganization and reality distortion, and examined whether these would be characterized by different patterns of cerebral

perfusion. The results showed that psychomotor poverty was characterized by reduced activity of the left dorsolateral prefrontal cortex (hypofrontality) and anterior cingulate. This provided support for the idea that negative symptoms are characterized by frontal lobe dysfunction. Patient scores on the disorganization factor showed reduced blood flow in the right prefrontal cortex, together with reduced activity of a left temporal lobe region involved in speech production. Lastly, reality distortion scores were positively correlated with blood flow in the hippocampal region, and left prefrontal cortex. Other studies have reported similar findings (Wolkin et al, 1992). For example, Schroder et al (1995) found that prefrontal glucose metabolism was associated with negative symptomatology, and delusions were associated with reduced activity in the hippocampus. McGuire et al (1993) studied a group of patients with schizophrenia while they were experiencing hallucinations, and later when their symptoms had remitted. Using SPECT, the hallucinatory state in the patients was characterized by increased blood in the left inferior frontal cortex, left temporal lobe and anterior cingulate. Given that medication may affect rCBF, Sabri et al (1997) studied a group of drug-naïve patients, and reported that thought disorder was associated with increased blood flow in frontal, cingulate and parietal regions, with severity of delusions and hallucinations

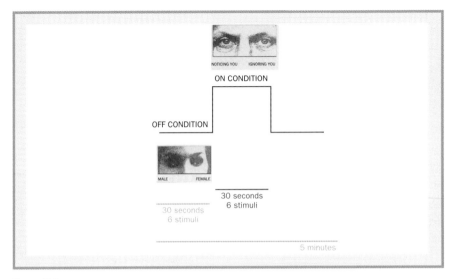

Figure 10.2
Eyes task of Baron-Cohen. Baron-Cohen et al, 1999. (Diagram courtesy of Tamara Russell.)

characterized by reduced blood flow in frontal, temporal and cingulate regions.

Liddle et al (1992) argued that symptoms of reality distortion (such as auditory hallucinations) are due to a failure of self-monitoring (Frith and Done, 1988), such that inner speech (thought) is not recognized as such, but instead is seen as 'alien' (McGuire et al, 1995). Given that these resting-state studies found that symptoms of reality distortion were associated with abnormal brain activity in frontal and temporal lobe regions related to language, McGuire et al (1995) suggested these symptoms may reflect abnormal monitoring of speech. Further support for this idea came from McGuire et al

(1995), who compared patients with schizophrenia with a history of auditory hallucinations with non-hallucinators, and observed that when asked to imagine another person speaking a sentence, the hallucinators failed to activate temporal and frontal regions, both activated by non-hallucinators and controls. In another study, McGuire et al (1996) studied rCBF when subjects with psychosis were producing thought-disordered speech in response to pictures. The results showed that thought disordered speech was positively correlated with blood flow in the parahippocampal region, and the right caudate nucleus. Thought disorder was negatively correlated with blood flow in the

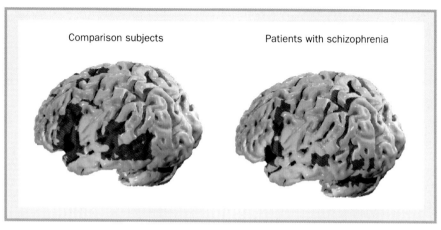

Figure 10.3
Generic brain maps of activation in comparison subjects and patients with schizophrenia during attribution of mental state to photograph of eyes. (View of the left hemisphere. Voxel-wise probability of type 1 error = 0.0004). Permission pending from Am J Psychiatry. *Russell et al, 2000.*

left and right inferior frontal gyri, left superior temporal gyrus and cingulate gyrus, again implicating abnormal activation of language areas of the brain.

In a study with exciting implications for the study of brain function in schizophrenia, Spence et al (1998) carried out repeat PET scans using $H_2^{15}O$ on a group of patients during an acute phase, and subsequently when they were in remission. Spence et al found that the patients had reduced activity of the dorso-lateral prefrontal cortex (DLPFC) at baseline (when psychotic), but that after 4–6 weeks when symptoms were improving, they showed increased blood flow in this region. This suggests that hypofrontality is a **state** rather than

a **trait** phenomenon. This finding has subsequently been replicated by Erkwoh et al (1999) using SPECT, who found that remission of active symptoms was associated with increased rCBF in frontal and temporal regions.

The notion of hypofrontality described above, has become a central theme of functional imaging research in schizophrenia. The original study by Ingvar and Franzen (1974) was followed by a large number of resting-state studies suggesting reduced frontal activity (Andreasen et al, 1997), probably linked to negative symptoms (Wolkin et al, 1992). Subsequently, studies have moved on from resting-state assessment to examine cerebral blood flow during performance of a cognitive task. Although the literature is contradictory, there is evidence to show that hypofrontality in schizophrenia is not merely a resting state phenomenon, but is reflected in reduced activation of frontal regions during task performance (Andreasen et al, 1992; Carter et al, 1998).

Functional imaging in schizophrenia has been used to study overall function during the resting state, and also to map cognitive functions and symptoms directly to brain regions and circuits, in the hope of identifying those regions and circuits which may be abnormal in schizophrenia. fMRI research into auditory or visual hallucinations – a common positive symptom of schizophrenia – has found that some of the brain regions linked to these hallucinations are also involved in 'normal' seeing and hearing processes. For example, Howard et al (1997) conducted a study of a man with Lewy body dementia who experienced persistent visual hallucinations. Researchers performed fMRI whilst shining light at the patient during, and in the absence of, continuous visual hallucinations. When he was not hallucinating, light stimulation produced a normal bilateral activation in striate cortex (part of the visual cortex). During hallucinations, very limited activation in the striate cortex could be induced, indicating that at least part of the activity in the brain responsible for the experience of visual hallucinations is located in the primary visual cortex. In an fMRI study of auditory

hallucinations, Woodruff et al (1997) found these were associated with reduced activity in brain regions that overlap with those that normally process external speech (temporal cortical regions). This is consistent with the idea that auditory hallucinations 'compete' with external speech for processing sites within the temporal cortex. The findings may explain why listening to music or speech helps to alleviate hallucinations in some people.

However, studies investigating the neurobiological basis of subsyndromes have primarily used resting state metabolism/perfusion as the dependent measure, which may overlook important functional cerebral deficits in response to cognitive processing. A recent fMRI study from our group characterized the patterns of functional cerebral response to cognitive load associated with schizophrenic subsyndromes. One hundred patients with schizophrenia were recruited for factor analysis of symptoms from clinical ratings. From this group, a subset of 30 patients and an additional group of 27 healthy volunteers underwent fMRI scanning during the performance of three cognitive paradigms, including verbal working memory, semantic categorization and a psychomotor task. The patients' factor scores from the clinical ratings were then regressed on to the fMRI data. Factor analysis revealed five latent factors including negative, positive, excited, cognitive and depressed subsyndromes. Regression of factor scores on to fMRI data revealed correlations with functional response specifically during the working memory condition, but not the other tasks. Severity of illness, indicated by summed factor scores correlated with functional response in several brain regions associated with language processing. Between-group comparisons revealed hypofrontality in the working memory task, and no differences for the other tasks (Honey et al, in press). This study showed that symptoms that co-occur in patients with schizophrenia are associated with distinct patterns of functional cerebral response, which is dependent on the nature of the cognitive task used to elicit activation. These findings provide some explanation of the inconsistencies evident in neuroimaging studies in schizophrenia.

Visualizing cognitive dysfunction in schizophrenia

Functional imaging research has now moved away from looking at schizophrenia as resulting from abnormalities in one or two regions – a lesion model – to looking at changes in neural circuitry. From their study of drug-naïve patients with schizophrenia, Andreasen et al (1997) concluded that the abnormal distribution of decreased and increased blood flow reflects a number of dysfunctional circuits that result in *'impairment of the ability to set priorities, process and produce information, and to turn it into*

meaningful thoughts and behaviour. This imbalance in circuits is expressed as psychotic or negative symptoms.'

The notion of **functional dysconnectivity** as it has become known, is now a central theme in neuroimaging research. Wiser et al (1998) studied rCBF using radiolabelled water ($H_2^{15}O$) during a memory task, and reported that despite equal task performance between patients and controls, the two groups activated different circuits to perform the task. The results showed that patients performed the task with significantly smaller increases in blood flow to the inferior, middle and medial frontal cortex, and left cerebellar cortex compared to controls. Compared to controls, patients had increased blood flow to the anterior cingulate, right superior temporal gyrus and fusiform gyrus. Wiser et al argue that the reduced blood flow in the prefrontal cortex and the cerebellum support the idea of **cognitive dysmetria** (Andreasen et al, 1998), which they define as *'a disruption of the interaction between cortical (especially frontal) functions such as initiation of memory retrieval or working memory, and cerebellar functions such as timing and sequencing, leading to "cognitive misconnections" and a disruption of the fluid co-ordination of mental activity.'* They argue that abnormalities in fronto-thalamic-cerebellar circuits provide an explanation of both positive and negative symptoms.

Functional dysconnectivity may provide an explanation for many of the symptoms and cognitive deficits associated with schizophrenia, however, debate continues about the circuits that are abnormal. Further evidence for functional dysconnectivity has come from a study by Jennings et al (1998). They also used PET scanning of regional brain activity during a semantic processing task. They used a technique known as path analysis with which it is possible to study how a change in activity in one region affects activity in the region to which it projects. From this, Jennings et al (1998) showed that regions which were positively connected in controls, i.e. increased activity in one led to increased activity in the other, were negatively connected in the patients with schizophrenia. In particular, abnormalities were seen in connections between frontal and temporal regions, and between frontal regions and the anterior cingulate. They also showed that regions where blood flow did not differ between patients and controls also had abnormal functional connections in the patients with schizophrenia. Abnormalities in connections between frontal and temporal regions and the cingulate have been supported by other studies (Fletcher et al, 1999)

fMRI studies of cognitive function in schizophrenia

Recently there has been increasing interest in cognitive dysfunction in schizophrenia, perhaps with the realization that cognitive

function and not necessarily psychotic symptoms might be related to functional outcome in schizophrenia. The functional imaging literature on mapping cognitive dysfunction in schizophrenia is very large and thus some representative studies are summarized in the chapter.

Previous studies have shown that schizophrenics consistently perform worse on tests of verbal fluency. This has been replicated in fMRI studies (Yurgelen-Todd et al, 1996; Curtis et al, 1998). Curtis et al (1999) investigated the extent to which hypofrontality may be a task-specific phenomenon. Having observed hypofrontality with verbal fluency, they investigated patterns of regional activation during a semantic decision task. The results showed that compared to controls, the patients with schizophrenia did not exhibit hypofrontality, however they did demonstrate higher levels of activity bilaterally in the fusiform and lingual gyri, and in the right inferior temporal gyri. These results again suggest that normal task performance in schizophrenia is still accompanied by abnormal patterns of brain activation.

Another domain where patients with schizophrenia often show impairment is in working memory. This obviously has major implications for normal daily functioning. Stevens et al (1998) found that while controls showed increased activity in the left inferior frontal gyrus, this activation was greatly reduced in the patients with schizophrenia during both verbal and non-verbal working memory tasks. Reduced activation was also observed in some temporal lobe regions. Together with the findings of structural abnormalities in the inferior prefrontal cortex (Buchanan et al, 1998), these results strongly implicate this region in the cognitive deficits and symptoms associated with schizophrenia.

The Wisconsin Card Sorting Test (WCST) is a test of executive function that is commonly used to demonstrate prefrontal dysfunction in schizophrenia (see Chapter 5). Volz et al (1997) examined regional brain activation during performance of the WCST in patients with schizophrenia using fMRI. The results showed that patients with schizophrenia made significantly more errors than controls, and exhibited significantly less activation of the right prefrontal cortex, together with increased activation of left temporal regions. This is yet more evidence for hypofrontality in schizophrenia, and the authors suggest that increased left temporal lobe activity may reflect '... *abnormal cerebral co-ordination* ...' – abnormal connectivity.

A frequent question is whether patients with schizophrenia exhibit cognitive abnormalities due to chronicity of the illness. O'Ceallaigh et al (submitted) used fMRI to determine whether abnormal patterns of cerebral activation previously detected in chronic schizophrenia are also present in the first episode. They compared brain function

in first episode and chronic schizophrenia during a verbal working memory task in which first episode and chronic patients were matched respectively to two groups of controls – first episode patients – control group 1, chronic patients – control group 2. There was no significant difference in activation pattern between the first episode group (controls–patients) and the chronic group (controls–patients). Abnormal patterns of cerebral activation in first episode schizophrenia are similar to those in chronic schizophrenia. This study showed that previously detected abnormalities in chronic schizophrenia cannot therefore be solely ascribed to psychosis symptomatology, long-term exposure to antipsychotics, or to post-onset disease progression.

Another interesting area in schizophrenia research has been the realization that social cognition may play an important role in the disease (see Chapter 7). A recent study used fMRI to investigate the hypothesis of a dysfunction in brain regions responsible for mental state attribution in schizophrenia (Russell et al, 2000). Median brain activation in patients diagnosed with schizophrenia was compared to that of healthy comparison subjects matched for sex and age during performance of a task requiring the correct identification of the emotional expression of a series of eye pairs. Patients showed reduced activation in left hemispheric inferior frontal and middle temporal brain regions compared to controls. This was the first study to show a neurocognitive deficit in a left fronto-temporal network in schizophrenia in association with impaired mental state attribution.

Patients with schizophrenia have problems in learning routine activities. This is important for functional outcome. Procedural learning (PL) is a type of rule-based learning in which performance facilitation occurs with practice on task without the need for conscious awareness (see Chapter 3). Impaired PL is found in patients with Parkinson's disease, Huntington's disease, cerebellar degeneration, prefrontal damage, and in schizophrenic patients on conventional antipsychotics. This study represents the first attempt to explore procedural learning deficits in patients with schizophrenia using fMRI. fMRI was used to acquire data during a sequence learning task in patients with schizophrenia on conventional antipsychotics and healthy normal subjects (Kumari et al, 2001). Normal subjects showed significant PL, but as expected, patients did not. In normal subjects, PL was associated with cerebral responses in the striatum, thalamus, cerebellum, precuneus, medial frontal lobe, cingulate gyrus and sensorimotor regions. No regions, except the anterior inferior gyrus, were significantly activated in patients. These findings support the previous literature in showing involvement of the striatum, cerebellum, thalamus, cingulate gyrus, precuneus, and sensorimotor regions in PL. Further fMRI studies with patients with schizophrenia receiving atypical antipsychotics which produce less dopamine-blockade in the striatum may help to establish whether impaired PL in this clinical population mainly reflects the effect of conventional antipsychotics via altered striatal activity. Other studies of neuroimaging the results of treatment in schizophrenia are presented in Chapter 15.

References

Andreasen NC. The role of the thalamus in schizophrenia. *Can J Psychiatry* 1997; **42**: 27–33.

Andreasen NC, Rezai K, Alliger R et al. Hypofrontality in neuroleptic-naive patients and in patients with chronic schizophrenia. Assessment with xenon 133 single-photon emission computed tomography and the Tower of London. *Arch Gen Psychiatry* 1992; **49**: 943–58.

Andreasen NC, Paradiso S, O'Leary DS. 'Cognitive dysmetria' as an integrative theory of schizophrenia: a dysfunction in cortical-subcortical-cerebellar circuitry? *Schizophr Bull* 1998; **24**: 203–18.

Baron-Cohen S, Ring H, William S et al. Social intelligence in the normal and autistic brain: an fMRI study. *Eur J Neurosci* 1999; **11**: 1891–8.

Callicott JH, Ramsey NF, Tallent K et al. Functional magnetic resonance imaging brain mapping in psychiatry: Methodological issues illustrated in a study of working memory in schizophrenia. *Neuropsychopharmacology* 1998; **18**: 186–96.

Carter CS, Perlstein W, Ganguli R et al. Functional hypofrontality and working memory dysfunction in schizophrenia. *Am J Psychiatry* 1998; **155**: 1285–7.

Copolov D, Crook J. Biological markers and schizophrenia. *Aust NZ J Psychiatry* 2000; **34**: 108–12.

Curtis VA, Bullmore ET, Brammer MJ et al. Attenuated frontal activation during a verbal fluency task in patients with schizophrenia. *Am J Psychiatry* 1998; **155**: 1056–63.

Curtis VA, Bullmore ET, Morris RG et al. Attenuated frontal activation in schizophrenia may be task dependent. *Schizophr Res* 1999; **37**: 35–44.

Erkwoh R, Sabri O, Willmes K et al. Active and remitted schizophrenia: Psychopathological and regional cerebral blood flow findings. *Psychiatry Res* 1999; **90**: 17–30.

Fletcher P, McKenna PJ, Friston KJ et al. Abnormal cingulate modulation of fronto-temporal connectivity in schizophrenia. *Neuroimage* 1999; **9**: 337–42.

Frith CD, Done DJ. Towards a neuropsychology of schizophrenia. *Br J Psychiatry* 1988; **153**: 437–43.

Honey GD, Bullmore ET, Sharma T. De-coupling of cognitive performance and cerebral functional response during working memory in schizophrenia. *Schizophr Res*, in press.

Howard R, David A, Woodruff P et al. Seeing visual hallucinations with functional magnetic resonance imaging. *Dement Geriatr Cogn Disord* 1997; **8**: 73–7.

Ingvar DH, Franzen G. Distribution of cerebral activity in chronic schizophrenia. *Lancet* 1974; **2**: 1484–6.

Jennings JM, McIntosh AR, Kapur S et al. Functional network differences in schizophrenia: a rCBF study of semantic processing. *Neuroreport* 1998; **9**: 1697–700.

Johnstone EC, Crow TJ, Frith CD et al. Cerebral ventricular size and cognitive impairment in chronic schizophrenia. *Lancet* 1976; **2**: 924–6.

Kumari V, Gray JA, Honey GD et al. Neural correlates of procedural learning: An fMRI study in normal and schizophrenic subjects. *Schizophr Res*, in press.

Liddle PF, Friston KJ, Frith CD et al. Patterns of cerebral blood flow in schizophrenia. *Br J Psychiatry* 1992; **160**: 179–86.

Longworth C, Honey G, Sharma T. Science, medicine, and the future: Functional magnetic resonance imaging in neuropsychiatry. *BMJ* 1999; **319**: 1551–4.

McGuire PK, Shah GM, Murray RM. Increased blood flow in Broca's area during auditory hallucinations in schizophrenia. *Lancet* 1993; **342**: 703–6.

McGuire PK, Silbersweig DA, Wright I et al. Abnormal monitoring of inner speech: a physiological basis for auditory hallucinations. *Lancet* 1995; **346**: 596–600.

McGuire PK, Silbersweig DA, Murray RM et al. Functional anatomy of inner speech and auditory verbal imagery. *Psychol Med* 1996; **26**: 29–38.

O'Ceallaigh S, Honey GD, Bullmore ET et al. Neural dysfunction in first episode and chronic schizophrenia during a verbal working memory task. Submitted.

Russell TA, Rubia K, Bullmore ET et al. Exploring the social brain in schizophrenia: left prefrontal underactivation during mental state activation. *Am J Psychiatry* 2000; **157**(12): 2040–2.

Sabri O, Erkwoh R, Schreckenberger M et al. Altered relationships between rCBF in different brain regions of never-treated schizophrenics. *Nuklearmedizin* 1997; **36**: 194–201.

Schroder J, Wenz F, Schad LR et al. Sensorimotor cortex and supplementary motor area changes in schizophrenia. A study with functional magnetic resonance imaging. *Br J Psychiatry* 1995; **167:** 197–201.

Spence SA, Hirsch SR, Brooks DJ, Grasby PM. Prefrontal cortex activity in people with schizophrenia and control subjects. Evidence from positron emission tomography for remission of 'hypofrontality' with recovery from acute schizophrenia. *Br J Psychiatry* 1998; **172:** 316–23.

Stevens AA, Goldman-Rakic PS, Gore JC et al. Cortical dysfunction in schizophrenia during auditory word and tone working memory demonstrated by functional magnetic resonance imaging. *Arch Gen Psychiatry* 1998; **55:** 1097–103.

Volz HP, Gaser C, Hager F et al. Brain activation during cognitive stimulation with the Wisconsin Card Sorting Test – a functional MRI study on healthy volunteers and schizophrenics. *Psychiatry Res* 1997; **75:** 145–57.

Wiser AK, Andreasen NC, O'Leary DS et al. Dysfunctional cortico-cerebellar circuits cause 'cognitive dysmetria' in schizophrenia. *Neuroreport* 1998; **9:** 1895–9.

Wolkin A, Sanfilipo M, Wolf AP et al. Negative symptoms and hypofrontality in chronic schizophrenia. *J Arch Gen Psychiatry* 1992; **49:** 959–65.

Woodruff PW, Wright IC, Bullmore ET et al. Auditory hallucinations and the temporal cortical response to speech in schizophrenia: a functional magnetic resonance imaging study. *Am J Psychiatry* 1997; **154:** 1676–82.

Yurgelun-Todd DA, Waternaux CM, Cohen BM et al. Functional magnetic resonance imaging of schizophrenic patients and comparison subjects during word production. *Am J Psychiatry* 1996; **153:** 200–5.

Conventional antipsychotic medications and cognition in schizophrenia

11

The discovery of the antipsychotic effects of chlorpromazine was a medical and scientific landmark of a magnitude comparable to the discovery of penicillin. Psychotic symptoms, in schizophrenia and other conditions, are remarkably responsive to treatment with these medications, to an extent comparable to the effectiveness of most 'successful' treatments in other domains of medicine. After the introduction of these medications in the 1950s, there was an exodus of patients from long-stay psychiatric treatment. While the living conditions for many of these patients was not good and the follow-up care provided to them ranged from absent to inconsistent, the fact that many of these patients experienced a remission of their psychotic symptoms for the first time in years was a truly remarkable thing. Enhancing the miraculous appearance of these symptom improvements was the fact that previously there had been essentially no treatments available that had any efficacy. As a result, within 15 years of the introduction of these treatments, the population of long stay psychiatric hospitals was reduced by two thirds (Wyatt, 1991).

Psychotic symptom reduction, in response to treatment with conventional antipsychotic medications, has been reported to be as high as 90% at the time of the first psychotic episode (Robinson et al, 1999). Rates of response to these treatments decrease across successive psychotic episodes, to the extent that the rate of treatment non-responsiveness to conventional medications can approach 30% in patients with an established course of illness (Kane et al, 1988). At the same time, 70% of patients still manifest substantial symptomatic reduction with treatment. Studies of spontaneous remission of psychotic symptoms conducted before the introduction of these medications suggested that about 30% of patients with schizophrenia manifest some improvement in their symptoms without treatment (Huber et al, 1975). Thus, the relative response rate, correcting for patients who would remit without treatment, is about 60% at the time of the first episode. Since some patients with a spontaneous remission of symptoms at the time of their first psychotic episode will never have symptoms or receive treatment again, it is more difficult to estimate what proportion of patients with schizophrenia would improve without treatment at later episodes. In any case, the odds that a psychotic patient with schizophrenia will experience moderate or greater reduction in their symptoms with conventional antipsychotic treatment are quite high.

Strengths of conventional medication treatment

There are several beneficial aspects of treatment with conventional antipsychotic medications. Patients who receive treatment with medication shortly after the initial episodes of psychotic symptoms tend to have a better overall lifetime outcome (Wyatt, 1991). While there are some failures to find that the 'duration of untreated psychosis' (DUP) predicts later overall outcome (Ho et al, 2000), these failures were often from studies whose patients had a duration of untreated illness that could be measured in months. Studies that compared patients who were untreated for years, such as patients studied at the time of introduction of these medications and patients from environments where the introduction of these medications were delayed, and contrasted their outcome to that of patients who received treatment within a few months of the development of their psychotic symptoms have found more consistent results (Quinn et al, 2000). Additional benefits of conventional medications include reduction of violent behavior and improvements in the quality of life of the caregivers of patients. There is little disagreement that these medications are quite effective in the reduction of psychotic symptoms.

Disadvantages of conventional medication treatments

Several major disadvantages of treatment with older medications have emerged over time. Both long-term (tardive dyskinesia, TD) and short-term (extrapyramidal symptoms, EPS) side effects are quite common in patients treated with these medications. Some of these side effects are irreversible and can cause long-term morbidity and mortality on their own. As many as 60% of patients with schizophrenia who receive treatment over a lifetime with conventional antipsychotic medications will develop TD and the initial incidence of this treatment in older patients is close to 15% per year (Jeste et al, 1999). Many patients do not understand that they are ill and their subjective experience of the illness and its treatment is more oriented toward the side effects of the treatment than its potential benefit on their illness. As a result, compliance with these medications is often poor and many patients are placed on long-acting (i.e. decanoate) treatments to enhance compliance. A considerable number of patients who are compliant with their treatment with these medications still experience exacerbations of their psychotic symptoms. Negative symptoms (e.g. flat affect) are much less improved with conventional antipsychotic treatments, compared to the efficacy of these medications on positive symptoms. Finally, as noted

above, a substantial minority of these patients develops a pattern of nonresponse to treatment over time (Lieberman, 1999).

A second disadvantage of conventional treatments is the need to use anticholinergic medication to reduce EPS and other parkinsonian side effects. While the use of these medications clearly reduces the severity of EPS and related features, there are several significant problems with these medications. Anticholinergic medication treatments have been shown to be associated with poorer performance on tests of memory (Strauss et al, 1990). Patients treated with these medications show a dose dependent failure in secondary memory functions, with a relative sparing of long-term memory. Attentional deficits are also noted in some patients. Older patients with schizophrenia who are treated with the combination of typical antipsychotic medication and anticholinergic medications have been reported to be markedly more impaired in their global cognitive functioning than patients treated with typical antipsychotic medication alone (Davidson et al, 1995). It appears, however, that the magnitude of memory impairment uniquely associated with anticholinergic medication is much smaller in patients with schizophrenia than it would be if healthy individuals were treated with these same drugs. However, a very small change may have marked significance, since patients with schizophrenia start out with considerable memory deficits (see Chapter 3) and a relatively smaller worsening may have a much greater functional effect. As a result, since these medications typically require the use of an adjunctive medication to control side effects, memory impairments are related to the use of these medications.

Possibly the greatest limitation of older medications is that they do not appear to markedly improve the overall outcome of schizophrenia. The proportion of patients with schizophrenia who are able to function independently (sustain employment, independent residence, and reasonable social functions) did not markedly improve with widespread adoption of these medications compared to the time before their introduction (Hegarty et al, 1994). When shifts in diagnostic practices are considered (Cooper et al, 1972), it is revealed that the proportion of patients meeting criteria for independent functioning was not markedly greater in 1985, when conventional antipsychotic treatment was widely employed early in the illness, than in 1895. It should be noted that the level of skills required of an individual to sustain independent outcome in 1985 was clearly much greater than in 1895. There have also been marked shifts in both the overall cultural attitudes toward the mentally ill and in the level of intactness of families who might have previously provided more support. However, patients with schizophrenia do not appear to be keeping up with changes seen in western culture in general in the requirements for successful adaptive life functioning.

Cognitive change with conventional antipsychotic treatments

A possible reason for the lack of improvement in outcome associated with conventional antipsychotic treatments is related to the profiles of differential efficacy of these older medications. As noted in Chapter 7, the best predictor of functional skill level in schizophrenia is cognitive functioning, with negative symptoms also found to be important. The severity of psychotic symptoms appears to be much less strongly associated with overall functional outcome and the ability to perform specific functional skills. Positive symptoms are reduced much more than negative symptoms by treatment with conventional antipsychotic medications. This is also true of the relative effect of conventional medications on cognition compared to positive symptoms. One of the most consistent findings in the research literature in schizophrenia is that conventional antipsychotic medications have remarkably limited effects, beneficial or adverse, on cognitive functions in schizophrenia (Medalia et al, 1988; Spohn and Strauss, 1989).

Conventional antipsychotic medications do not have wide-ranging deleterious effects on cognition: this point was made in Chapter 2. More surprising is their general lack of effect, positive or negative. Studies using a variety of research methods, including open label and blinded designs, have yielded relatively consistent results. Among the areas least affected include executive functioning and memory, two of the most critical areas for adequate functional outcome. The lack of effect on these domains of cognitive functioning may be at the centre of the overall modest effect on outcome of conventional medications.

There are a number of methodological problems in studies of the cognitive effects of older medications. Many studies did not use random assignment and others allowed the use of adjunctive medications that might have confused the results (Blyler and Gold, 2000). Finally, almost none of the studies controlled for practice effects through the use of alternate forms of tests that were employed in repeated-measures designs. Yet, the majority of these methodological problems favored finding a positive effect of conventional medications relative to the comparator conditions. Despite a significant methodological bias in favour of positive findings, such findings are remarkably absent from the literature.

There is some evidence from methodologically sound studies that conventional medications improve some aspects of attentional functioning. For instance, several studies have shown that treatment with conventional antipsychotic medications reduced the level of distractibility seen in patients with schizophrenia, increasing their ability to focus on relevant stimuli and ignore irrelevant information in both auditory and visual modalities (e.g. Harvey and Pedley, 1989; Oltmanns et al, 1979). In addition, patients who were more distractible when medication-free were more likely to have greater reductions in their clinical symptoms after the initiation of conventional antipsychotic treatments (Serper et al, 1994). Attentional response to treatment in the first week predicted reduction in Brief Psychiatric Rating Scale (BPRS) scores at 4 weeks and patients with greater attentional impairments responded better, in terms of global severity of psychopathology to higher doses of antipsychotics than to lower doses. However, these particular attentional impairments have not been shown to be related to functional outcome in patients with schizophrenia. Thus, conventional medications appear to selectively enhance certain aspects of cognitive functioning that are not related to functional outcome.

More limited positive evidence is available regarding improvements in vigilance with conventional medications. While there are consistent results showing that conventional medications reduce distractibility, there are as many negative as positive results in the domain of vigilance and related attentional domains. Furthermore, no research has convincingly shown that the specific vigilance tests shown to predict outcome are impacted in a positive way by treatment with conventional antipsychotic medications.

Only a few aspects of cognitive functioning appear to be worsened by conventional treatment and these measures have also not been proven to be related to functional outcome. In particular, performance on some measures of motor speed appear worse in treated patients when compared to untreated patients. These impairments appear transitory and related to the process of adjustment to initial treatment with these medications. Interestingly, some studies have shown that treatment with conventional antipsychotic medications may have a complicated relationship with performance on tests of vigilance (Harvey et al, 1990a). For example, in the continuous performance test (CPT), a test of vigilance described in Chapter 6, target stimuli appear continuously on a computer screen or over headphones. Subjects typically are asked to monitor the information stream and execute a motor response (often a button press) when they detect a target stimulus. Thus, a medication that enhanced the ability to detect target stimuli might have its beneficial effects cancelled if it also caused interference with motor skills and reduced ability to respond when the target was accurately detected. Some research has suggested that this might be true, in that performance on tests of motor speed have been found to be associated with CPT

scores in patients who are receiving conventional antipsychotic medications (Earle-Boyer et al, 1991; Harvey et al, 1990a; Walker and Green, 1982). In unmedicated patients, no correlation between CPT performance and motor speed was found. Since unmedicated patients perform better on tests of motor speed and the same on the CPT as medicated patients, it is quite possible that the patients receiving conventional medications have actually improved in their attentional skills and ability to detect targets, with the improvement undetected because of medication-related interference with the motor skills required to respond when the target is accurately detected.

An additional area where conventional medications might exert a deleterious effect is that of learning new information with practice. Many different adaptive skills are learned with practice and experience. Some of these skills are simple motor skills, such as the ability to execute an uncomplicated motor act repeatedly, similar to the skills required in working on an assembly line. Others are more complex activities, which require sequencing of multiple simple acts, or learning a set of procedures to apply in solving problems. Several studies (e.g. Bedard et al, 1996) have demonstrated that treatment with conventional antipsychotic medications is associated with impairments in procedural learning (see Chapter 3), when compared to no treatment or treatment with newer

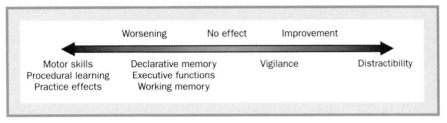

Figure 11.1
The gradient of effect.

antipsychotic medications. In addition, studies examining rate of learning of more complex skills, such as CPT performance, have yielded similar results. Finally, patients with schizophrenia who are tested repeatedly while being treated with conventional antipsychotic medications do not show the level of practice-related improvements shown by healthy individuals tested with the same tests (Harvey et al, 2000). As a consequence, one of the possible impairments induced by treatments with conventional medications may be subtle and impossible to detect at a single assessment, but critically important for functional outcome. Figure 11.1 demonstrates the hierarchy of influence of conventional medications on cognitive functions in schizophrenia.

The biological mechanism for lack of effect on cognition

All medications that are effective antipsychotics have effects on the dopamine D$_2$ receptor in the subcortical regions of the brain called the corpus striatum. No medication without these effects has ever been demonstrated to be effective at reduction of positive psychotic symptoms. Conventional medications also have multiple addition sites of action at neurotransmitters, including histaminergic, adrenergic, muscarinic (cholinergic), and other sites such as the sigma receptor and neuroactive peptides. In addition, the extent of dopamine binding per unit dose of the medication varies 50-fold or more, with medications referred to as 'high potency' or 'low potency' depending on their relative ratio of dopamine binding per dose (Keefe and Harvey, 1994). Most low potency medications also have more different sites of action than the high potency medications and, as a result, are more likely to cause sedation and related side effects. Despite a remarkable amount of clinical belief to the contrary, previous studies of the relative efficacy of older medications have demonstrated that once doses are equated for dopamine-binding potential, the effects of these medications on the clinical symptoms of schizophrenia are equivalent. Similar findings have evolved in terms of the lack of cognitive enhancing effects as well. There is no evidence that these medications, which vary widely in their secondary effects, vary in their ability to improve cognitive functioning in patients with schizophrenia. Thus, the secondary effects (adrenergic, muscarinic, histaminergic, etc.) are not the factors that lead to poor cognitive enhancement. The lack of enhancement must be due to some effect of these medications that is absent, some lack of effect on biochemical processes that would lead to enhancement of cognition.

It is somewhat easier to understand the impairing effects of these medications on motor speed and procedural learning. These are skills that require intact functioning of a variety of cortical and subcortical regions, including the basal ganglia. Since antipsychotics are also 'antidopaminergics', the induction of motor and procedural learning deficits can be partially understood on this basis. These cognitive symptoms are similar to those seen in idiopathic Parkinson's disease, a disorder of subcortical dopaminergic transmission. Similar to the reduced dopaminergic activity that is secondary to the death of dopamine neurons that occurs in Parkinson's disease, the shutdown of the subcortical dopamine system is the likely reason for these impairments in cognition

associated with conventional antipsychotic treatment. It may be that these side effects originate in the same transmitter tracts as EPS, which are also a symptom of Parkinson's disease and a consequence of irregularities in the level of transmission in the dopamine system.

Patients who are treated with conventional antipsychotic medications examined with positron emission tomography (PET) scans demonstrate increased metabolic activity in the striatum compared to unmedicated patients (Buchsbaum et al, 1992), with this increase caused by increased dopamine turnover due to the transmitter's inability to make contact with post-synaptic dopamine neurons. In contrast, cortical blood flow is not markedly increased in critical regions. As described in Chapter 10, decreased and poorly regulated cortical blood flow is a hallmark feature of schizophrenic patients when performing cognitively demanding tasks. Failure to increase and modulate this blood flow may be at the root of the failure of conventional medications to improve cognition in schizophrenia.

The fact that conventional medications offer markedly effective psychotic symptom relief but have no corresponding effect on cognition is not a paradox. Naturalistic studies of the relationship between positive symptoms and cognitive deficits, described in Chapter 2, have shown that there is essentially no correlation in the severity of these domains of illness. These findings hold in unmedicated patients, as well as in patients who are treated with conventional antipsychotic medications. In addition, patients whose psychosis has resolved, due to either treatment or spontaneous remission, have equivalently severe cognitive deficits (Harvey et al, 1990b). Thus, the complete lack of correlation, both with and without the perturbing effects of conventional medications on cognition, implicates different biological systems as the cause of these two domains of illness. The paradox, then, is not why the two domains do not respond in parallel to conventional antipsychotic treatment, but how one could possibly discover a treatment that could effect both of these domains at once. The next two chapters describe newer treatments that appear to have the potential to reduce both of these symptom domains at once.

Conclusion

Despite their markedly beneficial effects on psychotic symptoms, conventional antipsychotic medications are not effective in enhancing cognitive deficits in patients with schizophrenia. Cognitive impairments are not worsened, other than for motor skills, procedural learning, and practice-related improvements in skill learning. These impairments are similar to impairments seen in other conditions of subcortical dopaminergic underactivity, such as

Parkinson's disease. Since conventional antipsychotic medications, in order to control psychotic symptoms, reduce subcortical dopamine activity, the cause of both the clinical and cognitive adverse effects of these medications is probably related. Finally, most cognitive deficits are simply unchanged. We speculate that the reason that functional outcome in schizophrenia is not nearly as improved as the severity of positive symptoms is related to the lack of effect on cognition of these medications. As will be seen in the next two chapters, there may be a solution in the form of novel antipsychotic medications for schizophrenia and alternative pharmacological treatment strategies to enhance cognition.

References

Bedard MA, Scherer H, Delomorier J et al. Differential effects of D_2 and D_4 blocking neuroleptics on the procedural learning of schizophrenic patients. *Can J Psychiatry* 1996; 4: 21s–24s.

Blyler CR, Gold JM. Cognitive effects of typical antipsychotic medication treatment: another look. In: Sharma T, Harvey PD, eds. *Cognition in schizophrenia.* Oxford: Oxford University Press, 2000, 241–65.

Buchsbaum MS, Potkin SG, Siegel BV Jr et al. Striatal metabolic rate and clinical response to neuroleptics in schizophrenia. *Arch Gen Psychiatry* 1992; **49**: 966–74.

Cooper LE, Kendell RE, Gurland BJ et al. *Psychiatric diagnosis in New York and London.* London: Oxford University Press, 1972.

Davidson M, Harvey PD, Powchik P et al. Severity of symptoms in geriatric chronic schizophrenic patients. *Am J Psychiatry* 1995; **152**: 197–207.

Earle-Boyer EA, Serper MR, Davidson M. Harvey PD. Continuous performance tests in schizophrenic patients: stimulus and medication effects on performance. *Psychiatry Res* 1991; **37**: 47–56.

Harvey PD, Keefe RSE, Moskowitz J et al. Attentional markers of vulnerability to schizophrenia: performance of medicated and unmedicated patients and normals. *Psychiatry Res* 1990a; **33**: 179–88.

Harvey PD, Docherty NM, Serper MR, Rasmussen M. Cognitive deficits and thought disorder. II. An eight-month followup study. *Schizophr Bull* 1990b; **16**: 147–56.

Harvey PD, Moriarty, PJ, Serper MR, Schnur E. Practice-related improvement in information processing with novel antipsychotic treatment. *Schizophr Res* 2000; **46**: 139–48.

Harvey PD, Pedley M. Auditory and visual distractibility in schizophrenics: clinical and medication status correlations. *Schizophr Res* 1989; **2**: 295–300.

Hegarty JD, Baldessarini RJ, Tohen M. One hundred years of schizophrenia: a meta-analysis of the outcome literature. *Am J Psychiatry* 1994; **151**: 1409–16.

Ho BC, Andreasen NC, Flaum M et al. Untreated initial psychosis: its relation to quality of life and symptom remission in first-episode schizophrenia. *Am J Psychiatry* 2000; **157**: 808–15.

Huber G, Gross G, Schuttler R. A long-term follow-up study of schizophrenia: psychiatric course of illness and prognosis. *Acta Psychiatr Scand* 1975; **52**: 49–57.

Jeste DV, Lacro JP, Palmer B et al. Incidence of tardive dyskinesia in early stages of low-dose treatment with typical neuroleptics in older patients. *Am J Psychiatry* 1999; **156**: 309–11.

Kane J, Honigfeld G, Singer J et al. Clozapine for the treatment-resistant schizophrenic: a double-blind comparison with chlorpromazine. *Arch Gen Psychiatry* 1988; **45**: 789–96.

Keefe RSE, Harvey PD. *Understanding schizophrenia*. New York: Free Press, 1994.

Lieberman JA. Is schizophrenia a neurodegenerative disorder? A clinical and neurobiological perspective. *Biol Psychiatry* 1999; **46**: 729–39.

Medalia A, Gold J, Merriam A. The effects of antipsychotics on neuropsychological test results of schizophrenics. *Arch Clin Neuropsychology* 1988; **3**: 249–71.

Oltmanns TF, Ohayon J, Neale JM. The effect of medication and diagnostic criteria on distractibility in schizophrenia. *J Psychiatric Res* 1979; **14**: 81–91.

Quinn J, Moran M, Lane A et al. Long-term adaptive life functioning in relation to initiation of treatment with antipsychotics over the lifetime trajectory of schizophrenia. *Biol Psychiatry* 2000; **48**: 163–6.

Robinson DG, Werner MG, Alvir JM et al. Predictors of treatment response from a first episode of schizophrenia or schizoaffective disorder. *Am J Psychiatry* 1999; **156**: 544–9.

Serper MR, Davidson M, Harvey PD. Attentional predictors of clinical change during neuroleptic treatment. *Schizophr Res* 1994; **13**: 65–71.

Spohn HE, Strauss ME. Relation of neuroleptic and anticholinergic medication to cognitive functions in schizophrenia. *J Abnorm Psychol* 1989; **98**: 478–86.

Strauss ME, Reynolds KS, Jayaram G, Tune LE. Effects of anticholinergic medication on memory in schizophrenia. *Schizophr Res* 1990; **3**: 127–9.

Walker E., Green MF. Motor proficiency and attention-task performance by schizophrenic patients. *J Abnorm Psychol* 1982; **91**: 261–8.

Wyatt RJ. Neuroleptics and the natural course of schizophrenia. *Schizophr Bull* 1991; **17**: 325–51.

Novel antipsychotics as cognitive enhancers

12

Given the failures of typical antipsychotics in this regard as described in the last chapter, why would other drugs that reduce psychotic symptoms be expected to enhance cognition? In contrast to conventional antipsychotics, there appears to be considerable promise from these compounds for the enhancement of cognitive functioning. Recently, there have been a large number of studies done on the effects of these drugs on cognition in patients with schizophrenia. Although these studies have several methodological limitations, there is much to be learned from them.

The studies on cognitive enhancement in schizophrenia reflect one of the newest developments in the study of cognition in schizophrenia, with all of these studies published since 1993. These studies utilized a wide range of tests, with some using only a few neurocognitive measures and others conducting a more comprehensive neuropsychological assessment. The number of different neurocognitive tests included in each of the double-blind and open-label studies ranged from one to over 25. Test results from the cognitive assessments can be grouped into several categories presented in Table 12.1.

Four of the five randomized, double-blind studies reported

Table 12.1
Domains of cognitive function examined

1. Attentional processes
2. Executive function
3. Working memory
4. Learning and memory
5. Visuospatial functions
6. Verbal fluency
7. Motor speed
8. Fine motor function.

significant neurocognitive improvement on at least one measure following treatment with atypical antipsychotic medication compared to conventional antipsychotics. Seven of the nine open-label studies demonstrated improvement following treatment with atypical antipsychotics. Overall, 12 of 14 studies demonstrated improvement in some aspects of cognitive functioning compared to treatment with conventional antipsychotic medication. A meta-analysis of the studies published up to July 1998 found that, overall, the effects of these medications relative to conventional treatment was statistically significant (Keefe et al, 1999).

There are a wide variety of newer antipsychotic medications currently available in the US and worldwide. These medications have been available for variable periods of time, with clozapine re-introduced in the US in 1989, risperidone brought to market in 1994, and olanzapine, quetiapine, and ziprasidone introduced between 1996 and the

present. There are several other newer antipsychotic medications that will be brought to the market in the next 2 to 3 years as well. All of these medications have a number of similarities and differences, and all of these medications share the features of being serotonin-dopamine antagonists (SDA). The feature that they share with conventional antipsychotic medications is that they blockade the dopamine d-2 receptor. Medications that blockade the serotonin receptor without dopamine antagonism have proven ineffective as antipsychotics. Despite their common characteristics, these medications vary widely in several critical parameters. There is considerable variation in the extent to which they blockade other neurotransmitter receptors, including histamine, acetylcholine, norepinephrine, and other variants of the dopamine and serotonin receptors. In addition, the time course with which they blockade the dopamine receptors varies widely, with risperidone exerting the longest-lasting blockage and clozapine and quetiapine the shortest. Similarities between these medications in cognitive enhancing effects, therefore, are likely to be due to the combination of serotonin and dopamine blockade and differences, if any, are likely to be due to other aspects of neurotransmitter antagonism.

Studies have examined cognitive improvement following treatment with risperidone, clozapine, aripipazole (not yet on the market), olanzapine, quetiapine, and ziprasidone. The specific study results will be presented separately for the different compounds.

Results of drug studies

Clozapine

Treatment with clozapine has consistently been found to improve performance of patients with chronic schizophrenia on verbal fluency tests (e.g. Hagger et al, 1993). In addition, psychomotor speed and executive functioning have also shown improvements (Lee et al, 1994). These improvements appear to persist over time and increase with more extended treatment with clozapine (Buchanan et al, 1994). At the same time, in short term studies, clozapine appears to be associated with a slight worsening of performance on tests of visual memory and working memory. In studies of maze learning, clozapine was found to improve speed of performance compared to conventional antipsychotic medications (Lee et al, 1994).

The limitation of clozapine is that it is approved in the US only for use in treatment refractory patients, because of its potentially dangerous side effects. As a result, many patients would not be treated with this medication, despite its apparent benefits in certain aspects of cognitive functioning. In addition, the failures of clozapine to improve some aspects of memory or even to worsen memory performance must be considered in the context of the fact that most studies of this compound have been performed on a very treatment-refractory population with significant levels of cognitive deficit.

Risperidone

Treatment with risperidone has been reported to enhance executive functioning, as measured by maze learning (Meyer-Lindberg et al, 1997), trail-making test part B (McGurk et al, 1997) and the Wisconsin Card Sorting Test (Rossi et al, 1997) when compared to treatment with conventional medications. Patients treated with risperidone also manifested improvement in performance on selective attention and short-term memory (Green et al, 1997) as well as secondary memory when compared to patients receiving conventional treatments as well (Kern et al, 1999). These are important aspects of cognitive functioning in terms of the clinical predictors of functional outcome and the improvement effect was quite large. Other studies have shown that risperidone normalized reaction time performance (Stip and Lussier, 1996), improved motor skills (Kern et al, 1998), and enhanced the ability to recognize and perceive affects (Kee et al, 1998). One large-scale study (Harvey et al, in press) found that risperidone treatment enhanced memory, attention, executive functioning, and motor skills over an 8-week treatment trial. Finally, studies of the ability to learn skills with practice have shown that patients treated with risperidone were able to learn attentional skills with 4 weeks of practice to the point that these patients had performance that was significantly better than the baseline performance of healthy controls (Harvey et al, 2000a). Interestingly, as discussed in Chapter 11, patients treated with low doses of conventional medications showed no evidence of improvement with practice in this skill area.

Risperidone is the most widely studied of the newer antipsychotic medications. Results from studies with several different methods have found improvements, compared to treatment with conventional antipsychotic medications, suggesting that these improvements in cognitive functioning are not likely to be due to overall differences in treatment response, particularly of positive symptoms.

Olanzapine

This medication has been on the market for less time than risperidone and considerably less published information is available. In one study, olanzapine was associated with consistent improvements in cognitive functioning compared to conventional antipsychotic medications and, in some

analyses, relative to risperidone treatment as well (Purdon et al, 2000). In a much larger study, olanzapine demonstrated a substantial ability to enhance cognitive functioning compared to baseline treatment with conventional medications, but was no different in the magnitude of effect from risperidone (Harvey et al, in press). These areas of enhancement included executive functioning, attention, verbal memory, working memory, and motor speed. Clearly, much more research on this widely used medication will be appearing in the immediate future. The available evidence suggests that olanzapine is associated with wide-ranging improvements in cognitive functioning compared to conventional medications.

Quetiapine

This medication was initially slow to be adopted after its introduction, but is now more widely used. Only a few studies have been conducted with this medication. Treatment with quetiapine improved vigilance, as measured by the continuous performance test (Sax et al, 1998), and has been shown in a very small-sample study to be more effective than haloperidol across a wide array of cognitive measures (Purdon et al, 2001). A large number of studies on the cognitive enhancing effects of this medication are currently being conducted and the amount of information that is available will increase substantially in the near future.

Ziprasidone

This medication has been on the market for a matter of weeks at the time that this book was being written. As a result, there has been little research involving this compound to date. In a study examining selective attention and the continuous performance test (CPT), treatment with the novel antipsychotic medications ziprasidone and aripiprazole was associated with improvement in speed of response and in memory span (Serper and Chou, 1997). The number of subjects who were treated with each of those two medications was very small (n = 4) suggesting that these results should be considered preliminary only. In addition, a study examining the effects of switching patients who were doing poorly in the current treatment from conventional medications, risperidone, or olanzapine suggested improvements in executive functioning, attention, memory, and motor skills (Harvey et al, 2000b). This medication is also being studied with an extensive set of investigations. Much more data on this medication will be available soon.

The importance of these findings

Since cognitive impairment is correlated with the majority of the disability seen in chronic schizophrenia (Green, 1996; Green et al, 2000), treatment of this condition appears to have the potential to reduce this disability. Since the current group of novel antipsychotics has shown preliminary promise in this area, they may serve to improve the typically poor outcome seen in schizophrenia. There are several large-scale industry-sponsored trials that will go far beyond the initial preliminary studies. The industry-sponsored trials have large samples, double-blind methods, and comprehensive, conceptually selected assessment batteries. As a result, the findings of these trials will advance our knowledge far beyond where we are after examining these initial pilot studies.

There are many complexities in this area that will need to be resolved over time. The preliminary data are promising and for the first time suggest that medication for schizophrenia may improve the adaptive outcome of patients with this illness and increase quality of life in a way that far exceeds the improvements seen with typical neuroleptic medication. It will be important for the field to apply high methodological standards to the evaluation of the results of studies of cognitive enhancement in schizophrenia, in order to avoid unwarranted

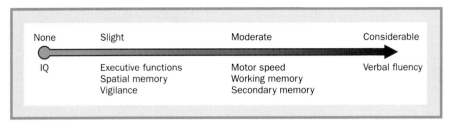

Figure 12.1
Changes in cognitive functions with newer antipsychotics.

optimism. In the next few years we will be able to come to an informed conclusion regarding the potential for cognitive enhancement with the new antipsychotic medications. If the early promise is realized, then major improvements in cognitive functioning and, possibly, overall functional status, of patients with schizophrenia may occur. Figure 12.1 shows the current status regarding cognitive enhancement with newer antipsychotic medications, presented in terms of which cognitive functions are more versus less well enhanced. Two important issues to keep in mind are the baseline level of impairment seen and the distribution of improvement scores. Most studies with adequate sample sizes have found that patients with the least baseline impairment show the most improvement. For example, patients whose baseline memory performance was impaired compared to healthy individuals but where the impairment was less than that typically seen in patients with schizophrenia were most likely to improve with treatment

(Harvey et al. in press). Patients with very severe impairments were least likely to improve. As a result, clinicians will need to be cautious in their expectations for change. Since many patients with schizophrenia have substantial impairments, some may not show marked benefits. It is important to realize that, similar to other symptoms of the illness, there may be variation across patients in the extent to which they improve with treatment.

Issues still to be addressed

There are several issues in cognitive enhancement with newer antipsychotics that have not been addressed, because of the relative newness of this whole research area. These issues are presented in Table 12.2. For instance, it is not clear if the optimal dose of newer antipsychotics with respect to control of psychotic symptoms is the same dose that would be maximally effective for cognitive enhancement. Dosing of newer antipsychotics has proven complex and several different

Table 12.2
Unresolved issues in cognitive enhancement

Dose response
Prediction of response
Magnitude of response
Rate of response
Implications of response

medications have had changes in their recommended doses for the control of psychosis. Essentially, no data are available with regard to whether the dose that is best for psychosis is the dose that is best for cognitive enhancement. While some studies have suggested that higher baseline performance predicts better response, these results are far from definitive. There are no data about other predictors of response, such as premorbid functions, age at onset, gender, education, or other factors that tend to be associated with clinical treatment response and with response to cognitive enhancers in the treatment of other conditions, such as attention deficit hyperactivity disorder (ADHD) or dementia.

The magnitude of response, in terms of average level of improvement for each of the cognitive content areas described above, is not well understood. There are relatively few studies and most of the studies have used different tests to measure concepts such as memory and attention. Some of the tests employed have very little information available about their reliability and validity,

meaning that failure to change with treatment may say as much about the test as the treatment. To this point, no study has suggested that any domain of cognitive functioning was improved to the point where the average performance of the patients with in the normal range, suggesting that there is no 'cure' yet for cognitive impairment.

An issue related to the magnitude of response, however, is the rate of response. If some proportion of patients are improving to a marked extent, while other patients do not change, then the average level of change would appear modest. Some of these patients, however, the ones with marked improvement, would be likely to experience a substantial benefit from this treatment. Unfortunately, most previous studies have not examined their data in this way and many studies had too few patients to even divide them into responders and nonresponders. Finally, most of the studies performed to date have not examined the correlates of cognitive deficits in schizophrenia: functional status and quality of life. It is possible, even in short-term studies, to examine changes in patients' perceptions of their life experiences. These data, as they become available later, will clearly provide substantial information regarding the importance of cognitive change. It is not currently known whether modest changes in cognitive functioning have an impact on quality of life that is greater than would be initially expected. If only large changes in cognitive functioning have important clinical implications, in terms of quality of life and functional change, then it is possible that only a subset of patients with schizophrenia will actually benefit from these treatments.

Differential effects of newer antipsychotic medications

Newer antipsychotic medications are quite diverse. While sharing a common SDA mechanism, they have multiple additional sites of action on dopamine, serotonin, noradrenergic, histaminergic, cholinergic, and NMDA receptor sites. It is conceivable that newer antipsychotic medications may have differential benefit on the cognitive symptoms of schizophrenia, possibly because of their secondary effects. Some of these effects might be beneficial and others might be adverse.

In terms of adverse effects, the secondary effects of conventional antipsychotic medications are as diverse as those of the newer medications, with no evidence of differential adverse effects. Even low potency medications that blockade cholinergic and histaminergic sites did not have adverse effects on cognition that could be distinguished from those of the higher potency medications that do not affect these neurotransmitter systems. In the domains of newer medications, both clozapine and olanzapine appear to blockade the cholinergic muscarinic receptors. Studies have reported that both of these medications,

and in particular olanzapine, enhance secondary memory performance (Harvey et al, in press). Enhancement of secondary memory is quite inconsistent with the effects of an anticholinergic compound, many of which have been shown to have marked adverse effects on secondary memory in schizophrenia. These data suggest, therefore, that some of the in vitro receptor affinities that have previously been measured are not particularly consistent with the in vivo effects of the compounds.

Very little current data support the notion of differential efficacy of newer antipsychotic medications. Extreme caution should be exercised in generalizing across different studies with different populations, different methodologies (i.e. blind vs. open; randomized vs. nonrandomized) and subtly different cognitive tests (Harvey and Keefe, 2001). Furthermore, there are common interpretive errors that occur when comparing across the results of clinical trials or across measures within clinical trials. For instance, a finding that compound A improves performance on a cognitive test from a baseline to a statistically significant extent while compound B does not, has no direct bearing on whether compound A is better at cognitive enhancement than compound B. If an improvement of 2.1 words in a word list learning test is statistically significant and 2.0 words is not, there is still very little difference between 2.1 and 2.0 words.

The only way to determine differences in cognitive enhancement, like differences in clinical response, is a 'head-to-head' study, one which compares the effects of two or more compounds in a methodologically sophisticated study with a large enough sample size to have power to detect differences. In addition, only a finding of a statistically significant difference in the change in scores from baseline across compounds has direct bearing on true differences in efficacy. So few of these studies have been completed that it is impossible to make any strong statements at this time. This is also an area where considerable new data will appear in the near future.

Limitations of these data

There are several limitations of some of the studies that have examined cognitive enhancement in schizophrenia with newer medications. Many of these studies completed to date do not meet minimum criteria for interpretable clinical trials, lacking random assignment, blinded assessments, and parallel study groups (Keefe et al, 1999; Harvey and Keefe, 2001). While these studies are truly preliminary, there may be limitations that interfere with the interpretability of the results. While most results from the methodologically less sophisticated studies have been replicated with better methods, some have not. As a result, it cannot be

determined exactly what the magnitude of effect of each of these medications would be in more sophisticated research designs.

Implications

This is one of the more important and most exciting domains of research on cognition in schizophrenia. If newer antipsychotic medications truly enhance cognition to a clinically significant extent, then a single treatment has the potential to improve all of the symptomatic aspects of schizophrenia and to improve outcome as well. The true test of cognitive enhancement with newer medications will be the upward modification of outcome. If these medications lead to change in functional outcome, then their effects go well beyond their originally noted benefits in domains of increased efficacy for positive symptoms and reduced side-effect profiles.

What if these medications do not lead to marked improvement for most patients? For the ones who are improved, even if they are not the majority, they are experiencing an improvement in their outcome that would not have happened with other medications. For the others, there is evidence that the use of additional cognitive enhancing medications, compounds that do not change clinical symptoms at all, can be safely accomplished in patients receiving treatment with newer medications. Since newer medications often do not require the use of anticholinergics, co-administration of drugs that enhance cholinergic functions is possible. Since most of these drugs have only modest other side effects, the cumulative side-effect burden will be less with these medications plus cognitive enhancers than with older medications plus cognitive enhancers. As described in the next chapter, the use of these additional cognitive enhancers is being studied in schizophrenia, with the possibility that even greater cognitive benefits can occur with the combination of stand alone cognitive enhancers plus newer antipsychotic medications.

References

Buchanan RW, Holstein C, Breier A. The comparative efficacy and long-term effect of clozapine treatment on neuropsychological test performance. *Biol Psychiatry* 1994; **36**: 717–25.

Green MF. What are the functional consequences of neurocognitive deficits in schizophrenia? *Am J Psychiatry* 1996; **153**: 321–30.

Green MF, Kern RS, Braff DL, Mintz J. Neurocognitive deficits and functional outcome in schizophrenia: are we measuring the 'right stuff?' *Schizophr Bull* 2000; **26**: 119–36.

Green MF, Marshall BD Jr, Wirshing WC et al. Does risperidone improve verbal working memory in treatment resistant schizophrenia? *Am J Psychiatry* 1997; **154**: 799–804.

Hagger C, Buckley P, Kenny JT. Improvement in cognitive function and psychotic symptoms in treatment-refractory schizophrenic patients. *Biol Psychiatry* 1993; **34**: 702–12.

Harvey PD. Effects of switching from conventional antipsycotics, olanzapine, or risperidone to ziprasidone. Presented at the American Psychiatric Association, 2000.

Harvey PD, Green MF, Meltzer HY, McGurk SR. The cognitive effects of risperidone and olanzapine in patients with schizoaffective disorder or schizophrenia. *Psychopharmacology*, in press.

Harvey PD, Keefe RSE. Interpreting studies of cognitive change in schizophrenia with novel antipsychotic treatment. *Am J Psychiatry* 2001; **158**: 176–84.

Harvey PD, Moriarty PJ, Serper MR, Schnur E. Practice-related improvement in information processing with novel antipsychotic treatment. *Schizophr Res* 2000; **46**: 139–48.

Kee KS, Kern RS, Marshall BD Jr, Green MF. Risperidone versus haloperidol for perception of emotion in treatment-resistant schizophrenia: preliminary findings. *Schizophr Res* 1998; **31**: 159–65.

Keefe RSE, Perkins S, Silva SM, Lieberman JA. The effect of atypical antipsychotic drugs on neurocognitive impairment in schizophrenia: a review and meta-analysis. *Schizophr Bull* 1999; **25**: 201–22.

Kern RS, Green MF, Marshall BD Jr et al. Risperidone vs. haloperidol on reaction time, manual dexterity, and motor learning in treatment-resistant schizophrenia patients. *Biol Psychiatry* 1998; **44**: 726–32.

Kern RS, Green MF, Marshall BD Jr et al. Verbal learning in schizophrenia: effects of novel antipsychotic medication. *Schizophr Bull* 1999; **25**: 223–32.

Lee MA, Thompson PA, Meltzer HY. Effects of clozapine on cognitive function in schizophrenia. *J Clin Psychiatry* 1994; **55**: 82–7.

McGurk S, Green MF, Wirshing WC et al. The effects of risperidone vs haloperidol on cognitive functioning in treatment-resistant schizophrenia: the trail making test. *CNS Spectrums* 1997; **2**: 61–8.

Meyer-Lindenberg A, Gruppe H, Bauer U et al. Improvement of cognitive function in schizophrenic patients receiving clozapine or zotepine: results from a double-blind study. *Pharmacopsychiatry* 1997; **30**: 35–42.

Purdon SE, Jones BD, Stip E et al. Neuropsychological change in early phase schizophrenia during 12 months of treatment with olanzapine, risperidone, or haloperidol. The Canadian Collaborative Group for research in schizophrenia. *Arch Gen Psychiatry* 2000; **57**: 249–58.

Purdon SE, Malla A, Labelle A, Lit W. Neuropsychological change in patients with schizophrenia after treatment with quetiapine or haloperidol. *J Psychiatry Neurosci* 2001; **26**: 137–49.

Rossi A, Mancini F, Stratta P et al. Risperidone, negative symptoms, and cognitive deficits in schizophrenia. An open study. *Acta Psychiatric Scandinavica* 1997; **95**: 40–3.

Sax KW, Strakowski SM, Keck PE Jr. Attentional improvement following quetiapine fumarate treatment in schizophrenia. *Schizophr Res* 1998; **33**: 151–5.

Serper MR, Chou JCY. Novel neuroleptics improve attentional functioning in schizophrenic patients. *CNS Spectrums* 1997; **2**: 56–60.

Stip E, Lussier I. The effect of risperidone on cognition in patients with schizophrenia. *Can J Psychiatry* 1996; **41** (Suppl. 2): 35S–40S.

Alternative pharmacological cognitive enhancers

13

As discussed in Chapter 12, newer antipsychotic medications improve cognition in some proportion of patients who are treated with them. At the same time, no study has shown that more than half of all patients manifest improvements that are substantial, suggesting that despite the improvements compared to conventional medications, the level of improvement is far from complete. As a result, alternative approaches may be required in order improve cognitive functioning, beyond the beneficial effects of newer antipsychotic medications.

Lessons from dementia

Dementia has long been defined as a condition where cognitive impairment is the cardinal feature. Studies of the progression of dementia have focused on the fact that adaptive impairments are correlated with the severity of cognitive deficit. In the case of progressive conditions such as Alzheimer's disease, Huntington's disease, and Parkinson's disease, progression of cognitive deficit precedes or co-occurs with the progression of adaptive deficit (Green et al, 1993). In contrast, 'behavioral' deficits are less systematically progressive and depression, agitation, delusions, and hallucinations occur in a widely distributed manner over the course of illness (Teri et al, 1989). Some evidence does suggest that psychotic symptoms in Alzheimer's disease occur with greater progression of cognitive impairment (Jeste et al, 1992), but that the severity of these disturbances does not always track progression of cognitive and adaptive deficits.

As a function of the primacy of cognitive impairment in dementing conditions, most treatment approaches for Alzheimer's disease have focused on cognitive enhancement. Many different compounds have been used for cognitive enhancement in Alzheimer's disease, with wide variation in the level of success of these approaches. Much can be learned from the methodologies employed in these clinical trials, including design issues, target populations, and cognitive and behavioral assessment strategies.

Critical cognitive enhancement issues

There are several critical questions to be addressed by cognitive enhancement studies in schizophrenia; these questions concern our understanding of the role of cognitive impairment in outcome and on appropriate clinical trials methodology. They address the issues of cognitive functioning over the lifetime, the role of the critical cognitive

functions that predict adaptive outcome, and the time-course of both cognitive enhancement and adaptive consequences of cognitive enhancement.

Which cognitive functions are improved? Are the critical outcome-related functions affected?

These may be the two most important issues in the treatment of cognitive deficits in schizophrenic patients. The studies reviewed in the last chapter suggest that several important cognitive functions may be improved following treatment with novel antipsychotics. Yet, the level of improvement is not associated with normalization of performance. Thus, selection of additional cognitive enhancers may require that they be targeted toward enhancement of these functions as well. Furthermore, since some cognitive abilities, such as verbal memory, vigilance, and executive functions, appear to be more strongly related to outcome than others, improvement in these areas is particularly important.

What is the timing of cognitive enhancement?

Time to onset

Some psychotropic compounds have immediate psychological and cognitive effects after administration and others appear to have a delayed course of action. For instance, amphetamine and related compounds have noticeable effects within half an hour of administration, while treatment with selective serotonin re-uptake inhibitors (SSRI) have a much more delayed effect on mood and related psychological processes. One of the critical issues in cognitive enhancement is understanding the latency to onset of cognitive enhancement effects, in order to identify adequate length of an effective treatment trial. Addressing this issue requires assessment of subjects immediately before and after initiation of treatment, as well as for a period of time afterward while receiving treatment with the potentially enhancing drugs.

Duration of enhancement effects

Most compounds affect cognition only while the drug is directly bioavailable and often only at a limited range of concentrations. As noted before, it has been argued that typical neuroleptic medication administered early in the course of illness leads to a better outcome (Wyatt, 1995), possibly by interrupting some neurodegenerative process. A compound that had such an effect on cognitive processes would also continue to exert an influence after administration was terminated. Thus, it may be possible that early treatment may cause cognitive enhancement through elimination

of a neurodegenerative process, although this interpretation is quite speculative at this time.

Are any improvements unique to the constructs of interest or are they due to generalized improvement of lower level functions (e.g. motor speed)?

Much of the research examining the association between outcome and cognitive impairment in schizophrenia has measured cognitive functioning with standard clinical neuropsychological tests. While this approach has the unambiguous benefit of using reliable and valid tests that are consistent in their administration across sites, these tests are multidimensional and adequate performance requires intactness of a variety of cognitive functions. It has been reported that the deficits of schizophrenic patients compared to normal individuals on the Wisconsin Card Sorting Test were accounted for completely by greater impairments on the part of patients with schizophrenia in working memory (Gold et al, 1997). It is also possible, for example, that a single cognitive process, such as information-processing capacity, could account for performance on all of these tests. It is further possible that improvements on these multifactorial tests could be accounted for by lower-level processes such as processing speed. This possibility has been raised before, where it was reported that all of the improvements in memory performance associated with tacrine treatment in a study of patients with Alzheimer's disease could be accounted for statistically by increases in reaction time performance (Sahakian et al, 1993). Thus, when interpreting cognitive enhancement effects, it is important to consider lower level processes, such as motor speed, that may be the actual factors that are improved.

Are there differing intervention strategies to be applied at different stages of the illness?

Acutely ill patients

Longitudinal studies suggest the most devastating clinical progression in patients with schizophrenia occurs within the first 5 years surrounding the time of onset (Ho et al, 1997). Episodes of psychosis in the early stages of illness may reflect an active pathophysiological process that can produce enduring cognitive and functional impairment in patients and reduce their capacity to respond to treatment (Lieberman, 1999). This model of the 'neurodegenerative' effects of psychosis in patients with schizophrenia suggests that the most debilitating effects of psychosis can be best limited by early, effective intervention. Thus, intervention with antipsychotics and additional cognitive enhancers in the early stages of schizophrenia may promote cognitive and functional

abilities later on in the illness. In addition, it is plausible that early intervention could have the potential to reverse some of the disability associated with the illness before it has secondary effects on the patient.

Cognitive enhancement with chronic patients

Since patients with chronic schizophrenia have established cognitive and adaptive impairment, it is possible that cognitive enhancement effects would have a different time course or magnitude in chronic patients as compared to first episode patients. First, since the cognitive impairments of chronic patients will be, on average, more severe than those seen in first admission patients (see Chapter 2) there may be a reduced enhancement effect in these patients and full recovery may not be expected. Second, it is unclear whether all cognitive deficits could be expected to resolve with the same time course. Similar to the possibility of secondary negative symptoms, there may be a process of secondary exacerbation of cognitive impairments associated with the experience of long-term deficiencies in cognitive functioning. For instance, if an individual has experienced impairments in attention and working memory that have persisted for years, other aspects of their cognitive functioning may be compromised because the component skills involved have never been exercised effectively. It may be expected that a period of adjustment to improvements in cognitive functioning would be required before other complex cognitive activities would be performed normally. Finally, a similar lag might be expected in the improvement in adaptive functioning associated with normalization of cognitive performance. If adaptive skills were ineffectively performed because cognitive impairments interfered with the ability to execute appropriate behaviors, then improvement might occur more rapidly than if a lifelong history of cognitive compromise had precluded effective learning of the skills in the first place. If new learning is required, then a longer time-course for improvement would be expected.

What compounds should be considered?

The most widely used and most effective cognitive enhancing medications used in psychiatry are amphetamines and related compounds. These medications are widely used in the treatment of attention-deficit hyperactivity disorder, in both children and adults, and have demonstrated consistent effectiveness for the treatment of cognitive deficits and the improvement of functional outcomes, including both school and work performance. These compounds have a primary effect on the dopamine system, but are active on the adrenergic system as well.

While these medications improve the aspects of cognitive functioning associated with outcome in schizophrenia, they are unfortunately not likely to be suitable for the treatment of patients with schizophrenia because of their potential to cause exacerbations of positive symptoms. At the same time, other agents with dopaminergic effects that lack the potential to worsen psychosis may be a promising strategy. Further evidence for the importance of the dopamine system has been provided by studies of dopamine metabolites, which are reduced in schizophrenia; this reduction is correlated with cognitive impairment (Berman et al, 1988; Kahn et al, 1994).

Compounds that enhance the functions of the cholinergic system also have promise for the treatment of cognitive impairments in schizophrenia. Cholinergic augmentation in animals enhances both secondary and working memory and has the potential to increase performance on tests of vigilance as well. Cholinergically active medications have been shown to have beneficial effects in both healthy individuals (Davis et al, 1978) and in individuals with cholinergic deficits, such as Alzheimer's disease (Rogers et al, 1996). Another major factor implicating the cholinergic system is the extremely high levels of smoking seen in patients with schizophrenia. Their level of smoking exceeds that of individuals in other western cultures by a factor of at least 3 to 1.

An additional domain of potential importance is the adrenergic system (see Friedman et al, 1999 for a detailed review). Compounds that specifically activate the adrenergic system have been shown in animal models to enhance working memory performance (Arnsten et al, 1988). Furthermore, these compounds have been shown to activate the regions of the anterior frontal cortex (Avery et al, 2000) that are inappropriately underactive in patients with schizophrenia (see Chapter 10 for a description). Finally, postmortem abnormalities in levels of adrenergic indicators have also been detected (Bridge et al, 1985). As a result, this specific transmitter system is a potentially important target for enhancement in schizophrenia.

Finally, the glutamate system is another potential target for cognitive enhancement (Krystal et al, 2000). This transmitter system interacts with the dopamine system and has been shown to be abnormal in postmortem studies of schizophrenic patients. In addition, compounds which influence the glutamatergic system have been shown to worsen both the symptomatic and cognitive features of schizophrenia and to produce schizophrenia-like cognitive impairments in healthy individuals.

While these four different transmitter systems have potential importance for the enhancement of cognition in patients with schizophrenia, the current level of knowledge regarding cognitive enhancement in schizophrenia in these domains is limited. The first reason for this limitation is that the recent focus on cognitive functioning as an important feature is a new one, with much of the prior research on augmentation therapy for schizophrenia focused on adding compounds to antipsychotic treatment with a goal of reducing refractory positive symptoms. The second reason is a much more practical reason: the availability of compounds that have these specific effects that are approved for use in humans. This second reason is related to the first: drug development has typically focused on development of antipsychotic medications which needed to have antidopaminergic effects as a primary mechanism of action. Little effort has been expended on the development of compounds which could be safely added to antipsychotic medications in order to enhance cognition.

Previous cognitive enhancement studies
Dopaminergic agents

For years there have been scattered reports of patients with schizophrenia demonstrating massive improvements following treatment with dopaminergic agents such as l-dopa or amphetamine. Patients most likely to respond to these treatments have been those with considerable negative or deficit symptoms and little in the way of positive symptoms. Concerns about worsening of symptoms have reduced these efforts to a trickle at the present time.

Recent studies have indicated that medications that have an agonist effect on the dopamine D_1 receptor improve spatial working memory in primates (Arnsten et al, 1994). In addition, administration of these compounds reverses haloperidol-induced memory deficits, with brief courses of agonist treatment reversing the effects of extended exposure to haloperidol in monkeys (Castner et al, 2000). Unfortunately, the most specific of these medications (SKF 38393) apparently does not reliably cross the blood–brain barrier. In primate studies, the compound is applied directly to the dopamine neurons in the anterior frontal lobe, leading to these marked improvements (Sawaguchi and Goldman-Rakic, 1994). Since hypoactivity of the D_1 system in the frontal lobes is a strong candidate for both the low level of elicited brain activity during cognitive demands and the actual cognitive deficits, the development of compounds that stimulate this system is a very high priority.

Cholinergic agents

These compounds have been studied for years as a potential treatment of Alzheimer's disease, which includes loss of cholinergic neurons as a central feature of the illness. Both direct cholinergic agonists for the muscarinic system (e.g. physostigmine) and compounds that indirectly increase activity by inhibiting the breakdown of acetylcholine by esterases have been employed. Direct muscarinic agonists have had relatively high levels of gastrointestinal side effects, despite their demonstrated efficacy in cognitive enhancement in both healthy and Alzheimer's disease populations.

In studies of schizophrenia, direct agonists were studied in the late 1970s and were noted to have effects on negative symptoms and tardive dyskinesia (Davis et al, 1976). No studies using contemporary diagnostic criteria have examined the effects of direct agonists. Several recent studies have examined the efficacy of cholinesterase inhibitors, specifically donepezil, on cognition in schizophrenia. While some of the open-label studies reported successful enhancement, the one double-blind trial found no overall effect (Friedman et al, in press). That study used patients with very severe cognitive impairment (typical memory performance of 4 standard deviations below normative standards) and found that there was a significant relationship between greater baseline memory impairments and failure to respond to treatment with donepezil. As a result, it is not clear whether there is a complete lack of promise or whether patients with more moderate impairments would benefit from treatment with cholinesterase inhibitors.

An additional issue is that of the differential effects of alternative cholinergic systems and potential cognitive enhancement. Although compounds that blockade the muscarinic nicotinic receptors can cause memory impairment, stimulation of the nicotinic system has been shown to have greater cognitive effects. While nicotine patch treatment has not shown marked promise in schizophrenia, smoking patients with schizophrenia have shown greater cognitive impairments when in nicotine withdrawal than when allowed to smoke. The next generation of cholinesterase inhibitors include one compound, galantamine, which directly stimulates the nicotinic receptors as well as reducing acetylcholinesterase activity. This compound may have more promise than the prior ones in enhancing cognition in schizophrenia.

Adrenergic agents

Studies with animals have indicated that the adrenergic 2_A agonist guanfacine enhances spatial working memory (Arnsten et al, 1994). Guanfacine has also been shown to increase blood flow to the anterior cerebral cortex (Avery et al, 2000). As noted in Chapter 10, this is the region that fails to activate under cognitive demands in patients with schizophrenia. In the one study to date on patients with schizophrenia (Friedman et al, 2001), this finding was confirmed, in that patients treated with the newer antipsychotic

risperidone plus guanfacine had better spatial working memory performance than patients treated with risperidone plus placebo. While this is only a preliminary study, the results are promising. Guanfacine did not have a generic activating effect and despite the fact that this compound is marketed as an antihypertensive, hypotensive side effects were not present. While more work is needed before this can be a recommended treatment, the combination of low incidence of side-effects and specific cognitive enhancement appears promising.

Glutamatergic agents

Glutamate is a complex neurotransmitter, the effective regulation of which appears critical for neuronal integrity. Glutamate has two receptor subtypes, the NMDA and AMPA variants. When a stroke occurs, the release of excess glutamate can cause neuronal death, while experimental manipulations that cause chronic glutamatergic underactivity in animals induces apoptosis, programmed cell death. Compounds that reduce glutamergic activity, particularly at the NMDA receptor, mimic schizophrenia (Krystal et al, 2000), including causing cognitive impairments that are similar to those seen in schizophrenia (Krystal et al, 1998). Glutamate is the most ubiquitous transmitter in the cerebral cortex, but its correct regulation appears more critical than that of any other transmitter in order to avoid dangerous consequences.

Glycine is a glutamate agonist that has been used to treat negative symptoms, with mixed results. Studies that have used higher doses have been more successful (e.g. Javitt et al, 1994). Studies have also shown that the administration of lamotrigine reverses the effects of the NMDA receptor antagonist ketamine (Anand et al, 1997). There have been no comprehensive studies on the effects of compounds that directly regulate glutamate on cognitive functioning in schizophrenia, but several studies have found modest beneficial effects on a limited cognitive battery (e.g. Goff et al, 1995). A considerable amount of work is currently aimed at development of compounds that normalize glutamate transmission with the goal of enhancement of cognition in schizophrenia.

Conclusions

Cognitive enhancement in schizophrenia with supplemental pharmacological treatment is an area that is sparking considerable current interest. The results of some small sample pilot studies have provided mixed results, with some evidence for success with adrenergic supplementation and less encouraging results for cholinesterase inhibitors and glutamatergic compounds. This area of major research and clinical interest is still in its infancy and new compounds are being developed all the time that might have applications in this area. There are several clear targets for later drug

development. The first is nicotinic stimulation. The second is dopamine D_1 agonists that can be used in humans. Third, and possibly most important, are the glutamatergic compounds that can be used to regulate glutamatergic activity in the cortex. As these drugs are developed and tested, there is likely to be an explosion of information in this domain of schizophrenia research.

References

Anand A, Chaney DS, Capiello A et al. Lamotrigine reduces the psychotomimetic, but not euphoric, effects of ketamine in humans. Conference presentation, Annual meeting of the ACNP, 1997.

Arnsten AFT, Cai JX, Goldman-Rakic PS. The alpha-2 adrenergic agonist guanfacine improves memory in aged monkeys without sedative or hypotensive side effects: evidence for alpha-2 receptor subtypes. *J Neurosci* 1988; **8**: 4287–97.

Arnsten AFT, Cai JX, Murphy BL, Goldman-Rakic PS. Dopamine D1 receptor mechanisms in the cognitive performance of young adult and aged monkeys. *Psychopharmacology* 1994; **116**: 143–51.

Avery RA, Franowicz JS, Studholme C et al. The alpha-2a-adrenoreceptor agonist, guanfacine, increases regional cerebral blood flow in dorsolateral prefrontal cortex of monkeys performing a spatial working memory task. *Neuropsychopharmacology* 2000; **23**: 240–9.

Berman KF, Illowsky BP, Weinberger DR. Physiological dysfunction of dorsolateral prefrontal cortex in schizophrenia. IV. Further evidence for regional and behavioral specificity. *Arch Gen Psychiatry* 1988; **45**: 616–22.

Bridge TP, Kleinman JE, Karoum F, Wyatt RJ. Postmortem central catecholamines and ante mortem cognitive impairment in elderly schizophrenics and controls. *Biol Psychiatry* 1985; **14**: 57–61.

Castner SA, Graham V, Goldman-Rakic PS. Reversal of antipsychotic-induced working memory defects by short-term dopamine D1 receptor stimulation. *Science* 2000; **287**: 2020–2.

Davis KL, Hollister LE, Barchas JD, Berger PA. Choline in tardive dyskinesia and Huntington's disease. *Life Sci* 1976; **19**: 1507–15.

Davis KL, Mohs R, Tinkelberg A et al. Physostigmine: improvement of long-term memory in normal volunteers. *Science* 1978; **201**: 272–4.

Friedman JI, Adler DN, Davis KL. The role of norepinephrine in the pathophysiology of cognitive disorders: potential applications to the treatment of cognitive dysfunction in schizophrenia and Alzheimer's disease. *Biol Psychiatry* 1999; **46**: 1243–52.

Friedman JI, Adler DN, Temporini HD et al. Guanfacine treatment of cognitive impairment in schizophrenia: A pilot study. *Neuropsychopharmacology* 2001; **25**: 902–9.

Friedman JI, Harvey PD, Adler D et al. Effects of donepezil on cognitive functioning and clinical symptoms in chronic schizophrenia. *Biol Psychiatry*, in press.

Goff DC, Tsai G, Manoach DS, Coyle JT. Dose finding trial of D-cycloserine added to neuroleptics for negative symptoms in schizophrenia. *Am J Psychiatry* 1995; **152**: 1213–15.

Gold JM, Carpenter C, Randolph C et al. Auditory working memory and Wisconsin Card Sorting Test performance in schizophrenia. *Arch Gen Psychiatry* 1997; **54**: 159–68.

Green CR, Mohs RC, Schmeidler J et al. Functional decline in Alzheimer's disease: a longitudinal study. *J Am Geriatr Soc* 1993; **41**: 654–61.

Ho B-C, Andreasen N, Flaum M. Dependence on public financial support early in the course of schizophrenia. *Psychiatr Serv* 1997; **48**: 948–50.

Javitt DC, Zylberman I, Sukin SR et al. Amelioration of negative symptoms in schizophrenia by glycine. *Am J Psychiatry* 1994; **151**: 1234–6.

Jeste DV, Wragg RE, Salmon DP, Harris MJ Cognitive deficits of patients with Alzheimer's disease with and without delusions. *Am J Psychiatry* 1992; **149**: 184–9.

Kahn RS, Harvey PD, Davidson M et al. Neuropsychological functioning correlates of central monoamine activity in schizophrenia. *Schizophrenia Res* 1994; **11**: 217–24.

Krystal JH, Belger A, Abi-Saab W et al. Glutamatergic contributions to cognitive dysfunctions in schizophrenia. In: Sharma T, Harvey P, eds. *Cognition in schizophrenia*. Oxford: Oxford University Press, 2000, 126–56.

Krystal JH, Karper LP, Bennett A et al. Interactive effects of subanesthetic ketamine and subhypnotic lorazepam in humans. *Psychopharmacology* 1998; **135**: 213–29.

Lieberman JA. Is schizophrenia a neurodegenerative disorder? A clinical and neurobiological perspective. *Biol Psychiatry* 1999; **46**: 729–39.

Rogers S, Doody R, Mohs RC. E2020 produces both clinical global improvement and cognitive test improvement in patients with mild to moderate Alzheimer's disease. *Neurology* 1996; **46**: A217.

Sahakian BJ, Coull JT. Tetrahydroaminoacridine (THA) in Alzheimer's disease: an assessment of attentional and mnemonic function using CANTAB. *Acta Neurologica Scandinavica* 1993, **88**: 29–35.

Sawaguchi T, Goldman-Rakic PS. The role of D1-dopamine receptor in working memory: local injections of dopamine antagonists into the prefrontal cortex of rhesus. *J Neurophysiol* 1994; **71**: 515–28.

Teri L, Borson S, Kiyak A. Behavioral disturbance, cognitive dysfunction and functional skill. Prevalence in relationship in Alzheimer's disease. *J Am Geriatr Soc* 1989; **37**: 109–16.

Wyatt RJ. Early intervention for schizophrenia: can the course of illness be altered? *Biol Psychiatry* 1995; **38**: 1–3.

Behavioral cognitive enhancement

14

The idea that cognitive functions can be enhanced through training in practice in schizophrenia is an old one. Following the 'practice makes perfect' model, patients with schizophrenia have been trained for years in cognitive skills, with modest success. While this area was not highly regarded a few years ago, some recent developments have preliminary promise for success.

The typical prior model for cognitive training or 'cognitive remediation' in patients with schizophrenia has always been repetitive practice. Patients were exposed to simple tasks and performed them repeatedly (Wexler et al, 1997). For instance, some cognitive remediation training would simply have patients perform tests such as the continuous performance test (CPT) for multiple trials (Benedict and Harris, 1989). Outcome measures would include whether performance on the primary task (the CPT) improved and also whether these results 'generalized' to other situations. While primary task performance would often improve, generalization was often poor (Brenner et al, 1996). Furthermore, when given a break in the training, performance on the part of schizophrenic patients would often return to its baseline level (Goldberg et al, 1987). These findings suggested that the short-term improvements seen were likely to be due to lower level factors, such as procedural learning, rather acquisition of more complex skills.

While this finding appears initially discouraging, the results of attempts to treat patients with head trauma or vascular accidents was essentially similar. Little progress has been made using models that simply offered repetitive practice. Recent training programs have increased in sophistication, with a slight improvement in the results. There are several components of these more sophisticated programs that are of interest. In addition, as seen in the last two chapters, both newer antipsychotic medications and alternative cognitive enhancers have demonstrated promise for the enhancement of cognitive deficits in patients with schizophrenia. As shown at the end of this chapter, the interaction between advances in medication treatment and more sophisticated skills training programs may lead to a large step forward in the results of cognitive remediation of patients with schizophrenia.

Structured problem solving training

One of the most difficult aspects of skill learning for patients with schizophrenia is the identification and incorporation of a strategy. When learning complex tests, patients with schizophrenia have a tendency to use random or trial and error problem solving. Several different strategies have been suggested to overcome these problems. As described elsewhere by Til Wykes (2000), these components have been presented as a single package, referred to as 'scaffolding'. This concept refers to the idea of building a stable problem solving structure for patients with schizophrenia by focusing instruction only on those aspects of performance where there is a problem, and making the steps that they take toward remediation slow, but sure.

One of the major problems in the structured approach to the treatment of patients with schizophrenia is the extreme challenges posed by these patients because of their difficulties in following guided instruction to improve their performance. For many years it has been known that patients with schizophrenia would fail to implement strategies that were suggested to them for improving their cognitive performance. Patients who failed to spontaneously notice the embedded semantic organization in lists of words that they were instructed to learn also failed to use the organizational characteristics of the list when the organization was pointed out to them at the beginning for the learning situation (Koh and Peterson, 1978). Even more extremely, patients with schizophrenia appear to benefit much less from some types of structured training than would be expected.

Several years ago, Goldberg et al (1987) presented the results of a failed problem solving training program as evidence that patients with schizophrenia had refractory lesions in the frontal cortex that rendered them unable to learn how to solve conceptual problems, regardless of training strategy.

In this study, patients with schizophrenia were presented with the Wisconsin Card Sorting Test (described in detail in Chapter 5). They were asked to perform the test, with the results being that the patients performed in a uniformly poor manner. They were then provided training, which included item-by-item instruction, with the correct responses provided to them along with the conceptual rationale for the correct response. During instruction, unsurprisingly, the patients' performance was markedly improved. Then another testing session was attempted, with the results being that the patients failed to show any carry-over from the extensive instruction that they had just received.

The results of this study led to a flurry of interest and controversy regarding the possibility of teaching patients with schizophrenia to perform the WCST. Obviously, if the typical patient with schizophrenia was unable to learn to perform this test with extensive training and feedback, the implications are quite negative. Performance on this test is strongly related to successful community outcome. If patients fail to show typical practice effects, then their prognosis for eventual independent living appears grim indeed.

Several other studies have found results that were more promising. In fact, training patients to perform the WCST was referred to as a 'cottage industry' (Goldberg and Weinberger, 1994). One of the positive consequences of this attention was the development of several different approaches to the training of patients with schizophrenia that resulted in promising gains in performance on this test.

Provision of conceptual models

One idea about why patients with schizophrenia have such a difficult time solving problems is that they have a difficult time with overall strategies. Giving conceptually oriented instructions at the outset of training has been shown to be associated with more rapid learning.

Trial-by-trial instruction

Provision of trial-by-trial guidance and feedback, rather than outcome-oriented feedback at the end of the task has been shown to increase the rate of skill learning. This strategy may overcome some of the memory problems that interfere with patients with schizophrenia patients learning across multiple trials.

Errorless learning

One hypothesis regarding the poor performance of patients with schizophrenia on cognitive tests is that they have initially poor performance and have been discouraged or demoralized, resulting in giving up too early (Kern et al, 1996). If the demands of the task can be adjusted in sequence, such that the patient never makes early errors, then they might have the potential to learn more rapidly. Some very recent data has substantiated this possibility.

Assessment of learning capacity

Some patients with schizophrenia improve in their WCST performance when trained with a program using the concepts described above. Those patients have also been shown to improve in several different domains after receiving training and instruction. Thus, one of the critical findings of the Goldberg study is that some patients with schizophrenia have truly limited capacity to learn with instruction, but others seem to have much more potential to benefit from instruction.

Factors that may influence ability to learn with practice

The hallmark of schizophrenia is variability and heterogeneity. This heterogeneity extends to response to cognitive rehabilitation. Many factors in schizophrenia are well-described but poorly understood, with variation in learning capacity being one of them. There are several factors that may influence response to rehabilitation, however.

Premorbid functioning

Patients with higher levels of premorbid attainment tend to perform better when receiving various types of training, including rehabilitation. This finding promises few intervention directions, however, because premorbid functioning is often correlated with intellectual functioning. Thus, finding that schizophrenic patients with lower IQs learn more slowly than individuals with higher IQs is not markedly different from what would be expected in the general population. However, one of the main reasons that patients with schizophrenia do not learn rapidly with rehabilitation may also be related to their baseline cognitive impairments.

Current cognitive functioning

As the rest of this book has clearly shown, many patients with schizophrenia have significant impairments in attention, memory, and rate of learning. It should be no surprise that these deficits have marked impact on skills learning. As this chapter has indicated, cognitive rehabilitation is a skills training procedure. This means that the more that a patient needs rehabilitation by virtue of having greater cognitive impairments, the less likely they are to receive notable benefits from rehabilitation interventions. As a result, patients with more severe current cognitive impairments appear to be the ones least likely to be able to learn new skills in structured training situations.

Medication status

As noted in Chapter 11, conventional antipsychotic medications fail to enhance cognitive functioning in patients with schizophrenia. In contrast, some benefit is noted from switching patients previously treated with older medications to novel antipsychotics. It may be that the switch to newer medications, combined with cognitive skills training, may lead to even greater benefits than either of the two alone.

In a recent study, the direct influence of type of medication (older/newer) on rate of skills learning was examined (Harvey et al, 2000). Patients randomized to treatment with either risperidone or conventional medications were given extensive practice in performing the CPT. Subjects were not provided with any instructions or feedback about their performance and there was no attempt to influence performance through any mechanism other than rote practice. As a result, this is a procedure that resembles older cognitive enhancement protocols, where

extensive rote practice provided a means of changing cognitive functioning. Similar to those older studies, the rate of improvement of patients treated with older medications and given extensive practice was negligible. Newer antipsychotic medication was associated with a notable improvement in performance. The two groups of patients did not differ in their baseline characteristics and did not differ in their performance at baseline, where both performed much more poorly than healthy comparison subjects. As shown in Figure 14.1, however, the patients treated with risperidone improved with practice to the point where their performance was significantly better than the performance of healthy individuals at baseline. In fact, their performance crossed the threshold for healthy controls after eight practice sessions.

This study did not examine generalization of skills to other performance situations and did not examine changes in outcome, and therefore its results must be considered tentative. The level of improvement seen, however, was much more rapid and complete than that seen in previous studies that used similar training methods, but with patients generally treated with older medications. Similar to studies of depression and attention deficit hyperactivity disorder, the benefit of behavioral and pharmacological interventions appeared to be larger than the result of either alone. Previous studies of the effect of risperidone treatment on CPT performance,

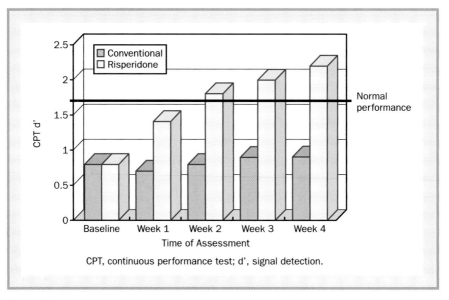

Figure 14.1
CPT performance as a function of type of medication.

without extensive training, has shown a much smaller effect. Training during treatment with older medications is associated with essentially no benefit. The implications are that more sophisticated training programs, those employing structured problem solving, errorless learning, scaffolding, and other strategies, in conjunction with newer developments in pharmacological treatments, may have the potential to have large and potentially generalizable effects.

Conclusions

Behavioral strategies for the enhancement of cognition have increased steadily in sophistication over the past two decades. Because of the employment of a variety of new strategies, behavioral cognitive remediation is poised for a breakthrough. Recent evidence suggesting that cognitive functioning can be enhanced in schizophrenia through the use of newer antipsychotic medications and through the use of supplemental add-on strategies has marked implications for behavioral cognitive enhancement. One of the effects may be essentially to raise the base level of schizophrenic cognitive performance. In particular, impairments in learning rate and attention that occur in neuropsychological testing situations are also found in cognitive remediation. Improving patients' ability to learn and pay attention through pharmacological therapy means that the results of training programs are quite likely to be improved as well. Similar to previous results regarding the combination of pharmacological and behavioral therapies, it is likely that the combination of pharmacological and behavioral cognitive enhancement will have greater results than seen in the past.

References

Bellack AS, Blanchard JJ, Murphy P, Podell K. Generalization effects of training on the Wisconsin Card Sorting Test for schizophrenic patients. *Schizophr Res* 1996; 19: 189–94.

Benedict RH, Harris AE. Remediation of attentional deficits in chronic schizophrenia patients: a preliminary study. *Br J Clin Psychol* 1989; 28: 187–8.

Brenner HD, Roder V, Hodel B et al. *Integrated psychological therapy for schizophrenic patients.* Gottingen (Germany): Hogrefe and Huber, 1996.

Goldberg TE, Weinberger DR. Schizophrenia, training paradigms, and the Wisconsin Card Sorting Test redux. *Schizophr Res* 1994; 11: 291–6.

Goldberg TE, Weinberger DR, Berman KF, Pliskin NH, Podd MH. Further evidence for dementia of the prefrontal type in schizophrenia? A controlled study of teaching the Wisconsin Card Sorting test. *Arch Gen Psychiatry* 1987; 44: 1008–14.

Green MF. Cognitive remediation in schizophrenia: Is it time yet? *Am J Psychiatry* 1993; 150: 178–87.

Harvey PD, Moriarty PJ, Serper MR, Schnur E. Practice-related improvement in information processing with novel antipsychotic treatment. *Schizophr Res* 2000; 46: 139–48.

Kern RS, Wallace CJ, Hellman SG et al. A training procedure for remediating WCST deficits in chronic psychiatric patients: an adaptation of errorless learning principles. *J Psychiatric Res* 1996; 30: 283–94.

Koh SD, Peterson RA. Encoding orientation and the remembering of schizophrenic young adults. *J Abnorm Psychol* 1978; 87: 303–13.

Wexler BE, Hawkins BA, Rounsaville B et al. Normal neurocognitive performance after extended practice in patients with schizophrenia. *Schizophr Res* 1997; 26: 173–80.

Wykes T. Cognitive rehabilitation and remediation. In: Sharma T, Harvey P, eds. *Cognition in schizophrenia.* Oxford: Oxford University Press, 2000, 332–51.

Functional neuroimaging of effects of antipsychotics in schizophrenia

15

There is a large body of evidence regarding the different pharmacological profiles of typical and atypical antipsychotic drugs, however, relatively little is known about their differential effects on cerebral function. Previous studies have shown that typical antipsychotic drugs are associated with increased volumes of basal ganglia structures (Chakos et al, 1994). One possible explanation for this is that it reflects increased blood flow in these structures. There is evidence from a positron emission tomography (PET) study to support this idea (Miller et al, 1997). The authors examined regional cerebral blood flow (rCBF) in a group of patients with schizophrenia while they were on typical antipsychotics, and subsequently after a 3-week drug-free period. The results showed that the patients with schizophrenia exhibited higher blood flow in the basal ganglia when medicated, compared to their drug-free state, together with decreased rCBF in frontal lobe regions. This supports the notion that medication-induced structural changes in the basal ganglia reflect vascular changes. Additionally, it shows that medication may be a confounding factor in studies that have found hypofrontality in schizophrenia.

However, functional Magnetic Resonance Imaging (MRI) is also becoming the technique of choice to visualize the

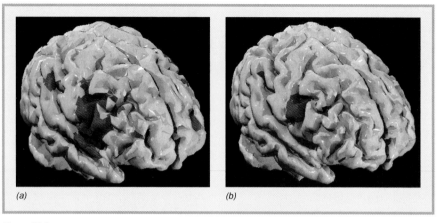

(a)   (b)

Figure 15.1
(a) Brain activity related to memory task in patients with schizophrenia showing lack of synchronised brain activity. (b) Specific areas of improved and synchronised brain activity with risperidone treatment.

dynamic changes in brain activity in response to drug treatment in schizophrenia. Such research may help resolve the debate among clinicians and healthcare providers on typical versus atypical medication, as these studies already point to marked differences in brain responses to these two types of antipsychotic drug (Stevens et al, 1998; Honey et al, 1999; Miller et al, 2001). Studies are beginning to use functional imaging to study the effects of different antipsychotic drugs on cerebral activity. The ability to monitor the effects of antipsychotic drugs on brain activity is likely to greatly aid our understanding of how drugs work, and help us to identify which drug would be most suitable for a particular patient (Figure 15.1).

The ability to conduct longitudinal

scanning has important clinical applications. Characterization of the functional neuroanatomy of cognitive processes will provide a framework for research investigating the longitudinal effects of pharmacological treatments on cognitive function. Research at our laboratory has followed pharmacologically induced changes in brain function as a result of switching patients with schizophrenia to newer atypical antipsychotics (Honey et al, 1999). This research raises the possibility of developing profiles of patients likely to respond well to particular drug treatments, so that the likelihood of positive treatment response can be assessed prior to embarking upon lengthy and expensive courses of treatment. It could also be used to develop treatment profiles outlining which disease-related cognitive deficits are enhanced by particular drug treatments. Another clinical implication of longitudinal scanning is that it enables fMRI to track changes in brain function, within individuals, over the course of an illness. For example, schizophrenia is characterized by a course of psychotic episodes and periods of remission. Longitudinal fMRI can be used to differentiate between neural deficits underlying the illness and those associated with exacerbation of symptoms during acute psychotic episodes.

In the study mentioned above, fMRI was used to study whether switching patients with schizophrenia from typical antipsychotic drugs to the atypical drug risperidone would produce differences in brain activity during a working memory task (Honey et al, 1999). Working memory deficits have been consistently reported in schizophrenia, and there is evidence of functional hypofrontality during working memory tasks (Stevens et al, 1998). Working memory performance has been shown to be related to prefrontal dopamine function (Watanabe et al, 1997), and given that there is evidence from animal studies that atypical antipsychotics increase prefrontal dopamine transmission (Hertel et al, 1996; Li et al, 1998), the authors predicted that switching schizophrenics from typical antipsychotics to risperidone would result in increased activity of prefrontal regions.

Patients were scanned at a baseline assessment when all were on typical antipsychotic drugs. Subsequently half of the patients with schizophrenia were switched to risperidone while the other half remained on their typical medication. Subjects were rescanned after 6 weeks. The results showed that patients switched to risperidone exhibited an increase in blood oxygenation in the right dorsolateral prefrontal cortex (DLPFC), precuneus and supplementary motor area (SMA) at follow-up. Risperidone restored fronto-parietal activation (noted in controls, but not in patients during the baseline) as compared to the activation seen at the baseline assessment, when the patients were on conventional antipsychotics. There was significantly greater change from baseline to 6 weeks in patients who were switched to risperidone than those who remained on conventional antipsychotics. The authors noted that the cause of the observed increased frontal cortical activity may reflect the effect of reduced D_2 receptor antagonism, reduced activity of inhibitory GABA neurons via serotonergic modulation, or alternatively serotonin-mediated increased frontal dopamine activity.

This shows that it maybe possible to 'reactivate' brain regions in psychiatric illness via drug treatment. The increased activation in prefrontal regions may help to explain improvements in cognitive functioning that have been observed with risperidone (Meltzer and McGurk et al, 1999), although it is important to note that in this study, increased cortical activation was not paralleled by significant improvement in task performance. This study also demonstrates the suitability of fMRI as a tool to assess psychopharmacological effects. Given that fMRI has many advantages for longitudinal study over techniques such as PET and single photon emission computed tomography (SPECT), this sort of approach could be used to study drug effects in other psychiatric disorders, such as the effects of cholinesterase inhibitors in Alzheimer's disease.

These data provided the first direct evidence of enhanced prefrontal and premotor function following substitution of risperidone for typical antipsychotics. It also highlights the potential value of fMRI as a tool for longitudinal assessment of the effects of new pharmacological treatments. In this instance fMRI has allowed researchers to demonstrate differences between the effects of drug treatments on brain regions involved in cognition. Future studies could also examine its utility in monitoring and evaluating neurobiological responses to psychosocial therapies such as cognitive behavioural therapy, which has shown promise in schizophrenia.

Conclusions

Structural and functional imaging studies have already revolutionized our understanding of the brain in schizophrenia and are continuing to provide further useful information. These

recent studies suggest that in the future, imaging may have a practical role in schizophrenia. However, the power of fMRI to track treatment changes and to provide more information about drug action may ultimately help to determine treatment choice in schizophrenia. A method of predicting treatment success would also allow patients to avoid the long and often unpleasant time that is currently necessary to see whether they are responding to treatment. Neuroimaging, in combination with other clinical, social, behavioural and cognitive techniques has potential as a useful biological marker for the detection and assessment of schizophrenia. While the clinical use of fMRI with schizophrenia is still some way off, its benefits – safety, resolution and speed – have led to exciting information about the illness and the effects of various treatment. It may ultimately prove a useful tool for determining treatment choices.

References

Chakos MH, Lieberman JA, Bilder RM et al. Increase in caudate nuclei volumes of first-episode schizophrenic patients taking antipsychotic drugs. *Am J Psychiatry* 1994; **151**: 1430–6.

Hertel P, Nomikos GG, Iurlo M, Svensson TH. Risperidone: Regional effects in vivo on release and metabolism of dopamine and serotonin in the rat brain. *Psychopharmacology (Berl)* 1996; **124**: 74–86.

Honey GD, Bullmore ET, Soni W et al. Differences

in frontal cortical activation by a working memory task after substitution of risperidone for typical antipsychotic drugs in patients with schizophrenia. *Proc Natl Acad Sci USA* 1999; **96:** 13 432–7.

Li XM, Perry KW, Wong DT, Bymaster FP. Olanzapine increases in vivo dopamine and norepinephrine release in rat prefrontal cortex, nucleus accumbens and striatum. *Psychopharmacology (Berl)* 1998; **136:** 153–61.

Meltzer HY, McGurk SR. The effects of clozapine, risperidone, and olanzapine on cognitive function in schizophrenia. *Schizophr Bull* 1999; 25: 233–55.

Miller DD, Andreasen NC, O'Leary DS et al. Effect of antipsychotics on regional cerebral blood flow measured with positron emission tomography. *Neuropsychopharmacology* 1997; 17: 230–40.

Miller DD, Andreasen NC, O'Leary DS et al. Comparison of the effects of risperidone and haloperidol on regional cerebral blood flow in schizophrenia. *Biol Psychiatry* 2001; **49:** 704–15.

Stevens AA, Goldman-Ravic PS, Gore JC et al. Cortical dysfunction in schizophrenia during auditory word and tone working memory demonstrated by functional magnetic resonance imaging. *Arch Gen Psychiatry* 1998; **55:** 1097–103.

Watanabe M, Kodama T, Hikosaka K. Increase of extracellular dopamine in primate prefrontal cortex during a working memory task. *J Neurophysiol* 1997; **78:** 2795–8.

Index